101 Handy Hints for a Happy Hysterectomy

By

Linda Parkinson-Hardman

Cover image © ROIM I Agency: Dreamstime.com

Published by: The Hysterectomy Association

www.hysterectomy-association.org.uk

ISBN 13: 978-0-9956957-2-6

Contents

This book is dedicated to everyone who had a part in creating this book, especially the many wonderful, vibrant and alive women who contributed through their own hints, tips and experiences.

Preface

This guide was originally created in 2005, and little about it has changed over the years. Different printers required different editions and this gave me the opportunity to rectify spelling or grammatical mistakes.

But, I had never revised the entire book; and it wasn't until a reader contacted me and said she found the book helpful and liked it because it was so *quaint*, that I realised it was long overdue for a major overhaul.

Reading through it was a little embarrassing, had I really bypassed the move to mobile phones and smart TV's; and thinking on some medicines and alternative therapies has changed in recent years too.

What you have in your hands is that major overhaul. Everything has been brought right up to date and some hints and tips have even been replaced altogether.

I hope the next generation of women who read the book find it as relevant for them as the others have done. I also hope that a lovely person in the future will also get in touch to let me know when this edition also becomes quaint.

Disclaimer

Although much of this book represents current medical opinion, some of the information and resources listed in this book are by definition, outside the scope of generally accepted medical standards of care. They may be non-conventional, alternative or complementary.

The information and resources listed should not be used in any way to provide a diagnosis or to prescribe any medical treatment. As in the case of conventional medicine, indiscriminate use of some therapies presented, without medical supervision may be harmful to your health. Individuals reading this material should in all cases, consult their own doctor or health practitioner for the diagnosis and treatment of medical conditions. The author and publisher cannot accept responsibility for illness arising out of failure to seek medical advice from a doctor.

Introduction

My own hysterectomy took place when I was 32; it changed my life. Before it, I was constantly ill, had serious problems with both endometriosis and IBS (irritable bowel syndrome) and would spend days every month in extreme pain. After it, I was suddenly well and I have never looked back, even though I couldn't have children.

But, I didn't know then, what I know now. I didn't know about the weight gain, the possible side effects of HRT, how tired I would be after the operation, when I could go back to work, what exercise I should (and shouldn't) do, and how much I would suffer from water retention. There were so many things I needed to know and there were so many things I could have done to make my recovery easier, but didn't.

What has always surprised me though is that even today, over 20 years on, I'm still being asked these same questions by the thousands of women who contact the Hysterectomy Association every year. 101 Handy Hints for a Happy Hysterectomy was written to answer this need. Hopefully it will provide you with some answers to the most common and frequently asked questions; as well as giving you some hints about how you can make your own recovery a successful one.

These hints will not give you all the information available; they are designed simply to raise your awareness so you can find out more about those that matter to you. Neither are they in any specific order of merit or importance, although they are loosely divided into five sections: preparing for hysterectomy, getting ready to go into hospital, now you're in hospital, recovery at home and long-term health. I would recommend reading through the whole book once and highlighting those you might like to go back to later.

This fifth edition has benefitted from the many personal questions, opinions, hints and tips I've received from women over the years through the Hysterectomy Association. The wonderful thing about receiving them is that I can see there really are common themes that have changed little, it's just the way of dealing with things might be different.

The Hysterectomy Association began life as a thesis for a Master's degree in Information Science. The women who took part in the research all asked for a source of information and support that was just for them. It has been running on a voluntary basis since 1997 and I hope you find the information in this book, and the others we publish, useful in helping you make some major decisions about your own future health.

Hysterectomy basics

Before we go any further, it's worth sharing some basic information about hysterectomy, including what it is and what it isn't.

Over 1.2 million women every year have a hysterectomy. Roughly 55,000 of those are in the UK. It is used to treat different gynaecological complaints such as fibroids, endometriosis, heavy bleeding and cancer. In most cases, a hysterectomy is 'elective surgery' this means that in most cases it is a choice that a woman has, rather than an emergency procedure. It can also be a surgery of last resort if there is uncontrolled bleeding following other surgery or even childbirth.

Hysterectomy is the surgical removal of the womb (uterus); this is known as a 'subtotal' hysterectomy. A 'total' hysterectomy also removes the cervix. And a 'total hysterectomy with BSO (bi-lateral salpingo-oophorectomy)' removes the womb, cervix, ovaries and fallopian tubes. It is important to remember that after having a hysterectomy you won't have any periods and you won't be able to have children.

There are two main ways to perform a hysterectomy. The most common is to remove the womb through a cut in the lower abdomen, usually along the bikini line. The second, less common, way is to remove the womb through a cut in the top of the vagina, the top of vagina is then stitched.

Most hysterectomies are performed when a woman is aged between 40 – 55, however many do occur before and after this age. Women who haven't yet gone through the menopause who have a hysterectomy that removes their ovaries, as well as other organs, will go through the menopause immediately following the operation regardless of their age, this is known as a surgical menopause.

Those who haven't gone through the menopause and have a hysterectomy that leaves one or both of their ovaries intact, have a 50% chance of going through the menopause within five years of their operation, again regardless of their age.

If you have your ovaries removed you may be prescribed HRT (hormone replacement therapy) depending on the reason you had your hysterectomy.

Recovery after a hysterectomy is a very personal experience which means your experience will be unique and unlike anyone else's. It is governed by a lot of factors that include how ill you have been leading up to your hysterectomy, how you react to anaesthetic, why you had your operation, what type of operation you had, your age, general fitness levels, how much support you have at home, the type of work you do and whether you have additional stressors to deal with (such as small children or dependent relatives). Of course, this list is not exclusive and there may be other additional factors to consider.

Preparing for Hysterectomy

Before you read any further, visit *www.hysterectomy-association.org.uk* and sign up for your free booklet and six weeks of daily recovery hints and tips. These are delivered to your email inbox from the day of your hysterectomy to help you through the first few weeks, and are different to the hints and tips you'll find in this book.

1. Be prepared and informed

Tom Lehrer, a mathematician from Harvard in the 1950's, wrote a somewhat degenerate song called Be Prepared[1].

> *If you're looking for adventure of a new and different kind*
> *And you come across a girl scout, who is similarly inclined*
> *Don't be nervous, don't be flustered, don't be scared*
> *Be prepared!*

Although the Boy Scout in question obviously had other, more risqué adventures in mind we can still learn from him. As you read through this book, you will be pointed to 'girl scouts' who are 'similarly inclined', and by sharing your knowledge and concerns, you will find you are less nervous, flustered and scared.

This is one time in your life when information counts and getting enough of it will depend on how much you already know. As we often say at The Hysterectomy Association, "you don't know what you don't know"; because of that simple fact, asking questions becomes difficult as health professionals assume you already know everything because you aren't asking questions - and so the loop goes around.

You've taken the first positive step by purchasing this book. These hints and tips will give you some ideas, but everyone is different and you will want answers to questions that are particularly relevant to your own set of circumstances, so you may find that some hints are more relevant than others.

Find some more good books, sign up for the daily hints and tips on the Hysterectomy Association website, join the forums, search the internet and ask other women about their experiences. But be aware, not all information is 'good' information and some can be positively 'bad'. As you read, listen for more questions to ask your doctor, and when you do get an answer don't forget to write it down.

2.   Start a journal

So, you're having a hysterectomy? Why is that; what has life been like since you started having health problems?

How has it affected your achievements, relationships and 'joie de vivre'? On the worst day you can remember, describe in a sentence how you felt. How did you feel when you woke up in the morning? How do you feel now? Describe what you want as an achievable goal for the day. What's your general state of health? How's the pain; can you give it a number between 1 and 10, with 1 being the least pain and 10, the most? Have you noticed anything that reduces the pain (lying down for example), or can you identify what made it worse?

And suddenly you're reading your journal entry for last Monday. And already, in just one week you can see you've come so far.

By keeping a daily or twice daily journal, not much more than a few notes jotted down through the course of the day, not only will you see you're having less pain, but you will feel more in control. After all, just look at your progress in the last week!

In the appendices of this book is an example page from our scaling diary, this is one way to track your recovery and record how you feel each day. If you send an email to *resources@hysterectomy-association.org.uk* you can request a free set of resources to download that accompany this book, including some scaling diary pages.

Alternatively, why not get one of the Hysterectomy Association's *My Hysterectomy Recovery Journal's*? It's ready to use immediately and full of extra hints and tips, recipes and resources you can use over the first six weeks of your recovery. Buy it on our website at *www.hysterectomy-association.org.uk*

3.   Find your support network

We all need help sometimes but one thing many of us aren't good at, is asking for help when we are having a hysterectomy; possibly because we're embarrassed about having problems with our 'lady bits' or we don't want to come across as needy. And yet, this is one of the most important ways we can help our recovery.

Your support network is going to be made of lots of people and might include your immediate family and friends; people you can call on or pay to do household chores and the school run; supermarket delivery services and maybe even social services if you live alone, are a single parent or are elderly and don't feel able to manage.

Everyone's support network is going to be unique as we all have different needs and priorities, so thinking about the type of help you might need and for how long is really important. One way of deciding on what your network might help with is to make a list of the various things you do in a 'normal' week. These might include working, shopping, ironing, cleaning, cooking, looking after children and caring for other relatives. Some of them you can disregard for the time being, like work, because you'll be taking time off to recover, but others will be on-going whatever your state of health.

You may also find that you need to plan well in advance for special occasions, such as Christmas and birthdays. Once you have your list, you can then think about how best to manage the activities and set up the right system to support you.

4.   Fill the freezer and your store cupboard

A woman once told me that when she had her hysterectomy the surgeon brought his patients into hospital on Sunday night and surgery was scheduled for the following Tuesday. He did this so they could have a rest because they were so tired from trying to get home and family organised.

Unfortunately, the NHS doesn't allow us the luxury of a couple of days of bed rest before surgery these days, and I suspect many of us feel we must make sure everyone copes while we're away. However, I have yet to talk to anyone who said their family went hungry because they hadn't filled the freezer before they had their hysterectomy.

There may be some virtue though, in organising yourself for when you get home from hospital, particularly if you live alone. A couple of weeks' worth of healthy frozen meals and weekly delivery of an organic farm box full of fruit and vegetables, should make even the most health conscious of us feel virtuous.

You may have already picked up the menus from all the takeaways that deliver in your area, or even found someone in the 'phone book that makes, and delivers, healthy nutritious meals. Even better would be training your partner and family not to assume you're going to disappear into a 'phone box, twirl round three times and emerge in a Superwoman outfit the very day you return from hospital!

5.   Stop smoking

Giving up, or cutting down, on your cigarettes if you are smoker is a 'no brainer' really. The risks of surgery are increased if you smoke because nicotine increases your heart rate and blood pressure. According to a joint briefing paper[2] from ASH (Action on Smoking and Health) and the Royal College of Surgeons of Edinburgh, the Royal College of Anaesthetists and the Faculty of Public Health smokers are 38% more likely to die after surgery than non-smokers.

Smokers also have an increased risk of lung and heart complications, post-operative infection, impaired wound healing (especially important for those women having an abdominal hysterectomy), require more drugs and longer stays in hospital, are more likely to end up in intensive care and increase their risk of emergency readmission. In fact, they state *"Smoking is the most important factor for the development of postoperative cardiopulmonary and wound-related complications in elective cases"*. As almost all hysterectomies are elective surgery, it's a point to take note of.

Doctors in Australia recommend quitting at least eight weeks before your surgery takes place, this gives your body time to adjust and start to recover.

6.　　Getting fit or fitter

This isn't really about losing weight; this is about making sure your body is in the best possible condition to undergo surgery. You might even find that getting fitter improves some, or all, of your symptoms.

What about improving your lung and heart capacity through some sort of aerobic exercise, just enough to increase your normal heart rate for 30 minutes three times a week. No, I'm not suggesting a Body Blitz workout, but why not put on some music and have a dance around the sitting room or take the dog (or yourself) for a walk every day.

Improving your diet, increasing your intake of water and walking a little every day will ensure your joints and muscles are in tip-top condition.

Exercise can also help to manage any pain you may have; it does this through the release of endorphins, the body's natural painkillers. Other ways to release endorphins include laughter, deep relaxation and reducing stress levels; these are all good ideas when you are about to have surgery don't you think?

7.　　Ditch the diet

If you're on a diet for weight loss now might be time to ditch the diet and change the way you eat instead. After all, 'you are what you eat' and if you eat junk food, your body won't be in the best condition to help you recover after surgery.

If you do have a little weight to lose, then changing the way you eat by cutting down on sugary drinks, cakes, biscuits, crisps and sweets, and increasing your fruit and veg intake will go a long way to creating a fitter, healthier you. Not only will you recover more quickly afterwards, but you will minimise the strain on your heart and other vital organs while you are anaesthetised.

An easy way to get the best out of your body, and your diet is to try and stick to the 'five a day' rule, eating at least five different portions of fruit and vegetables a day. A portion is roughly 80 grams and it's easy to incorporate them if you also link them to colours; red tomatoes, green peppers, oranges, purple sprouting broccoli ... the list is endless (almost).

If cooking all this seems like a chore, then why not use a juicer or blender, add your chosen pieces of fruit or vegetables in one go and drink your way to health; simple and effective.

8.   Explore your alternative options

In many ways, being offered a surgical intervention like hysterectomy can provide you with the motivation to take stock of your life and look at how lifestyle, diet and major events might have contributed to your current state of health.

Can you change the prognosis through your diet? Can you reduce your stress levels? Do you really need to have this surgery? You might be surprised at the number of medical conditions that seem to have poor diet, lack of exercise or stress as a contributory factor.

As well as improving your diet, increasing the exercise you take and reducing your stress levels, there are many complimentary therapies that may have a positive impact on your health.

Acupuncture for instance is a well-known method of pain management; reflexology and aromatherapy techniques can promote relaxation and could therefore help those conditions made worse by stress. Simply drinking more water can help flush toxins out of the body, and combining it with one of nature's anti-inflammatories and antiseptics such as Aloe Vera[3], which is reputed to heal both internal and external wounds, can be hugely beneficial.

9.   Face your fears

I get several emails every week from women saying they are anxious, nervous, worried and even frightened by their surgery. They are concerned that they are the only ones feeling like this, but it's normal to fear change; and major surgery, like a hysterectomy, is significant change.

The reason we fear it is because it's unknown. What can make it worse is that our fears can easily overcome us, especially as these are fears which aren't often talked about, or even admitted to, in many cases. But, it is surprising how much better you feel when you do confront what's bothering you by asking the questions you have about your hysterectomy as it will put them into perspective.

So, what are your fears?

Writing them down and admitting the worst you think can happen, can help you to prepare yourself physically, emotionally and mentally.

Try this exercise one day when you have an hour or two to yourself.

Gather together paper and pens and put them on a side table; then sit in your favourite chair and close your eyes. Imagine yourself in a beautiful garden, see the plants and flowers, smell the scents, touch the petals and slowly feel your body relaxing.

When you are fully relaxed open your eyes and think about the worst things that could happen because of your operation; write them down as they come into your mind and try not to analyse them before getting them down on paper.

Once you have written down as much as you can think of, close your eyes again, imagine the garden and slowly relax your body.

When you feel relaxed, open your eyes and read through the list you have written down.

Now think about what you can do to find out more about each of the things you have identified. This may involve talking to your GP, family and friends, it may involve research on the internet or at your local library, you could ask a question in the Hysterectomy Association forums and you might even be able to get in touch with your gynaecologist.

As you find out more information write it down, you will find in a very short time you feel more in control and the fears, although they may still be there, will become more manageable. At the same time, you will be less stressed and much calmer, in fact someone who finds it easier to recover from a hysterectomy.

Fear is often a fear of the unknown So banish the unknown with knowledge.

10.   Join a support group

There are many advantages to joining a support group of some description, including the fact that hysterectomy is not one of the most popular subjects to talk about over coffee at work! Sometimes it can be difficult to identify other women that have had one as they often don't want to talk about it - this is a shame as you can learn so much from other women's experiences.

However, despite these problems, there are many ways to get support from your fellow travellers. As hysterectomy support groups that meet up are few and far between, you may find it easier to join one of the many online forums. It's in these places you can ask the daftest and most personal questions and get encouraging, informative answers back.

The answers will come from a wide range of women from all over the world, who are just a few weeks or months ahead of you and who may have found a different way of managing your problem.

Most of these groups are free to join, have fantastic archives full of interesting conversations and you can just 'lurk' for a few days, weeks or months to see what is going on before plucking up courage and joining in. They also have the benefit that it may be a quicker way to get an answer than waiting to see your GP.

Why not try the Hysterectomy Association forums; find them online:

forums.hysterectomy-association.org.uk

11.   Ten questions to ask your gynaecologist

1. Have I had all the necessary diagnostic tests?
2. Why are you recommending a hysterectomy?
3. Are there any alternative treatments I could try first?
4. Do I need to have my ovaries or cervix removed, if so why?
5. What type of hysterectomy could I have; abdominal, vaginal or minimally invasive?
6. How long do you expect me to be in hospital?
7. Will I need to take HRT and what are the pros and cons?
8. What type of anaesthetic can I have?
9. What are the long-term consequences of having a hysterectomy?

10. What are the risks associated with a hysterectomy?

12.   Explore the alternative treatment options

These days it's much less common to be offered a hysterectomy than it once was. The reason for this is because there are so many other options that may alleviate or even get rid of the problem you have.

You may already have tried some of them in your journey towards surgery, but it's still worth asking if there's anything else to try first. The reason for this is that treatments change, new ones become available and others improve their success rates.

The availability of treatments depends on several factors including whether there is a practitioner in your area, if they are appropriate for your particular set of health problems and are licensed for use in the UK by NICE (National Institute for Health and Care Excellence).

The reasons you might consider an alternative treatment (if it is available) will be different for everyone, but they might include whether you have completed your family or not, whether you are prepared to try complementary medicine or if you are concerned about the possible increased risk of heart disease or osteoporosis if your ovaries are removed.

13.   Do I really need my ovaries and cervix removed?

Removal of the ovaries[4,5] and cervix[6,7] was, for a long time, a standard part of every hysterectomy in the UK. Fortunately, in recent years there have been changes in surgical techniques and attitudes, and this is much more likely to be a choice you make yourself, rather than being an assumption.

For many conditions, such as fibroids, heavy bleeding and prolapse there may be no medical reason to remove either the ovaries or the cervix and you should discuss your options with your gynaecologist.

If you are given a choice, it is worth bearing in mind that research is increasingly suggesting that their removal is not necessary if they are healthy and not involved in your medical condition.

The reason most commonly given recommending removal is that it helps prevent a possible problem in the future, however, unless you're at high risk of developing cervical or ovarian cancer then you may feel that while they are still healthy you will hang on to them. Of course, keeping your ovaries will mean that you won't have to consider the pros and cons of HRT immediately; and if you keep your cervix, then you will continue to need regular cervical smears.

If you do opt to have your ovaries removed, or if it's an essential part of your surgery then you will experience menopausal symptoms, even if you have already gone past the menopause. This is because the ovaries continue to produce small amounts of oestrogen for many years after we think they stop working.

If you haven't yet gone through the menopause, then removal of the ovaries will trigger the menopause within a short time.

If you have your cervix removed, either because you choose to or because of your health condition, then it may affect how intensely you experience orgasm after your hysterectomy. Although most women say that this isn't an issue, some women do report it as a side effect of the surgery.

If you do keep your ovaries it's important to know that in 50% of women under the age of menopause they fail earlier than they might have done, at least two years earlier and in some cases almost immediately.

If you start experiencing any symptoms that could be considered menopausal, you may want to talk to your GP about taking HRT, especially if you are still in your 30's or 40's.

14.   Start a question list

All the reading you do at this stage will help because it identifies concerns, worries and issues you hadn't thought about; a great source for these are other women's stories, and there are lots on the Hysterectomy Association blog. But, here's the thing, these are OTHER people's stories, they aren't yours. And, whilst they can shine a light on something you weren't aware of, you can't assume it will be the same for you.

I really believe that knowing as much as possible, the good, the bad and the downright ugly, is a positive thing for most women. The reason I believe this is because all the research shows if you know what could happen then you aren't as frightened or worried as if it came out of the blue. Other women's stories can tell you the absolute worst as well as the very best; the best thing about them is that they show these women coped, got through it and could write about it later.

So, when you are wandering around the web, reading stories and articles that alarm you, take out a notebook or download an app like Evernote or OneNote to your phone, and write the question down.

You can then check it out with someone who may know the answer; your GP, gynaecologist or a nurse are good starting points; women on the forums you use are another; they may say it'll never happen to you because of the surgery you're having or the health condition you suffer from. In other words, you'll be more knowledgeable about what to expect and why.

Whenever you think of a question note it down, then, when you see your doctor you can nonchalantly open the question list and stun him with your knowledge. Not only that but you can write the answers down to refer back to.

If you feel a bit nervous about asking your doctor all these questions take a friend or your partner along to appointments with you and they can make sure you ask all the questions and help you remember the answers.

15.   Will you need HRT?

You only need to think about taking HRT immediately after your hysterectomy if you are having your ovaries removed and have hadn't your menopause yet. Having your ovaries removed before you are 50ish will result in what's called a 'surgical menopause' and in some extreme cases, especially in younger women, it can begin in just 24 hours after surgery.

If you have already gone through your menopause and have your ovaries removed, you will almost certainly experience more menopause-like symptoms; this is because your ovaries were still producing tiny amounts of oestrogen, when they are removed this goes and the consequence is hot flushes, night sweats and all the other symptoms you thought were behind you. Of course, they won't be as bad as the first time around, but they will be noticeable.

There is no right or wrong decision to make as everyone is different so we have listed some of the pros and cons below; you may be able to add some more of your own to our list[8].

Why you might	Why you might not
high risk of osteoporosis	past the menopause already
high risk of heart disease	high risk of breast cancer
severe menopausal symptoms	high risk of thrombosis
age at hysterectomy	hysterectomy for endometriosis

If you have a hysterectomy and your ovaries are removed because you have endometriosis, then you may be advised not to take HRT for up to twelve months after your operation. This is because there is a risk that the replacement oestrogen contained in HRT will encourage a re-growth and therefore any endometriosis still left after surgery needs the opportunity to die off completely. After this time, you should be able to take it without any recurrence of the disease.

Finally, there is nothing to say you must take HRT; you could choose to use more natural ways of managing any menopausal symptoms, but more about those later.

Whether you then choose to take HRT will depend on your personal circumstances and attitudes. So, if you are over fifty, have already gone through the menopause and don't like the idea of taking drugs you may decide it's not for you. Alternatively, if you're in your late thirties you may feel you are simply replacing the hormones you would have continued to produce naturally for some time to come.

16.   Investigate testosterone supplements

If your ovaries are removed, not only will you lose oestrogen but you will also stop producing progesterone and testosterone.

Testosterone is vital for female wellbeing as small amounts are produced throughout your menstrual cycle and if you were to go through the menopause naturally, your ovaries and adrenal glands would continue to produce testosterone for up to twelve years.

In a woman, testosterone acts on mood and sex drive[9]; it can also provide relief from hot flushes and night sweats. Symptoms of testosterone deficiency can include lack of libido, having no energy and depression.

If you don't want to take testosterone, then supplementing with Zinc may help, as some studies[10] have shown that impotent men taking zinc supplements improved their potency and raised their levels of testosterone to normal.

Although there are no licenced testosterone treatments for women in the UK, it's worth talking to your GP about any concerns you have as they may still be able to prescribe something for you.

Getting ready for hospital

17.   Invest in a recovery cushion

It could be a favourite cushion from home, a comfortable pillow from your bed; you could even go out and buy or make a special one like the ones we sell on the website shop. It's something to cuddle while you're not well, you can even pop a heated (or cooled) gel pad in some.

Whatever you decide to use, you'll use it most days after your operation for lots of different things.

It'll be the most fantastic comfort blanket when you feel sad or fed-up, and it's something comfy to rest your feet on when you've had your daily dose of walking. You can hold it firmly against your tummy when you want to laugh or cough as it will support your aching muscles; and you'll be able to lie on your side with it stuffed under your tummy, providing just enough support until you get used to the very strange internal shifting and pulling feeling.

Finally, it's a favourite stuffed between you and the car seat belt as it stops it rubbing against the tender areas of your abdomen when you're a passenger in the car again.

If you are handy with a needle and thread, you could make your own recovery cushion, instructions are on the Hysterectomy Association website, you can find it by searching for '*Recovery Cushion*' in the search box on the home page.

18.   Buy a nightie

You may sleep naked at home, you may wear pyjamas, you may even wear an old tee-shirt. Whatever you wear at home, in the hospital you'll need a nightie, preferably cotton. It covers you up, allows surgeons and nurses easy access to check on any wounds you may have and it's cool.

Back at home, you may want to go back to what you've always worn, all or nothing; or you may prefer to carry on wearing a nightie for a few weeks; it won't let your wounds catch on anything and it won't be tight around the middle either.

Buy two or three (you'll want another to wear when you receive all those visitors and well-wishers when you get home).

Take your time over choosing the ones that say the most about who you are going to be once the operation is over and the recovery begins.

19.   The value of BIG knickers

There is no doubt about it, this is the one time in your life that you will really appreciate Big Knickers in a way you haven't done since you read or watched 'Bridget Jones's Diary'.

Your tummy muscles will be very tender for several weeks, and you really won't appreciate the area being rubbed by knicker elastic. If you have any wounds you will need to avoid them catching on lacy bits too.

For you, Big Knickers are going to be 'so this season', that you really need to invest in a few pairs before your hysterectomy.

Make sure that they come well up to your waist and aren't a size too small, this is no time for vanity ladies.

Under no circumstances think about going for a thong right now, they're going to be far too painful. Treat your tummy kindly and it'll repay you in a few weeks' time.

20.　Treat yourself to new scent

Sexy is one thing that many of us don't feel when we have a hysterectomy; but this is one area of our lives that could benefit the most with freedom from those awful symptoms. Preparing for the 'New You' takes some planning, and treating yourself to a new scent may be a good way to start.

Choosing a smell that makes you feel good acts on all sorts of senses, can stimulate happy feelings and invoke pleasant memories for each of us.

Together with new night wear, knowing we smell good could help us feel better even while we are still in hospital recovering. Some scents can even help the healing process by acting on the olfactory centres of the brain; these include lavender, myrrh, orange and ravensara.

But, if you do use a perfume, don't spray before the operation; and certainly, don't use it anywhere near any wounds after surgery, at least until you are all healed.

21.   Invaluable Arnica

My mother swears by Arnica and usually carries a small pack of ampules in her emergency first aid kit. This homeopathic preparation is often recommended by complementary therapists for physical and emotional shock. It is thought that arnica promotes healing, helps control bleeding and reduces swelling as the herbs' active ingredients are known to have mild pain-relieving, anti-inflammatory, and antibacterial actions[11].

It is an alpine plant, a member of the Compositae family and a relative of the common daisy. It contains selenium and arnica ash is rich in manganese. Both selenium and manganese are powerful anti-oxidants in the human body; in addition, manganese is an essential element needed for healthy bones, wound-healing, and the metabolism of proteins, cholesterol and carbohydrates. This accounts for the belief it may cut down the length of time it takes to recover after surgery. You can also use arnica cream on any abdominal or upper leg bruising, although you must avoid getting it on any open wounds or sores.

It used to be recommended that you took it, according to the instructions on the packaging, for three days before surgery and three days after. However, if you are thinking about taking it before surgery, please mention it to your gynaecologist and anaesthetist as there is a small risk of increased bleeding during surgery and it may influence how you are sedated. And do consult a homeopath if you are thinking of taking it for longer.

You can buy arnica from any good pharmacy. Although the homeopathic remedies are safe to use as they have been diluted many times, do not under any circumstances ingest the herb itself as it is highly poisonous.

22.   The importance of ritual

Ritual plays an increasingly minor role in our secular society, but it can be a very effective way of letting go emotionally so you can close a door on this chapter of your life.

The purpose of such a ritual is to prepare you emotionally, and perhaps mentally, for your hysterectomy by asking for help with the healing process and to acknowledge any loss you may feel. It also helps you to embrace the positive changes that the operation can bring into your life such as freedom from ill-health, pain, restriction and worry.

A ritual can be as simple as lighting a candle and saying a prayer; or it can involve friends and family who will be there to support you throughout your recovery period. The Hysterectomy Association has a ritual on the website and you can find it by typing the word 'ritual' into the search box. You are welcome to use or adapt for your own purposes.

23.   Buy a good book

As you won't be doing much of anything else, a good book can keep you absorbed for days, and you've already made a good start by buying 101 Handy Hints for a Happy Hysterectomy!

But seriously, what I'm really talking about is that list of books you keep intending to read because they've been recommended by friends or your book club. Why not go to the library, visit your local book shop, browse Amazon, or even check out your local charity shop.

Of course, you may prefer e-books to the physical variety, after all the latter take up valuable storage space. An e-reader, such as the Kindle or even its app can turn your phone, laptop or tablet into a 'book on the go', giving you the joy of keeping up with the story even while you're waiting in a queue.

For those who are visually impaired then e-readers can be a godsend, as they can often be used to 'speak' the book out loud. Alternatively, if you own a member of a library then you can probably download digital editions from their catalogues and even listen to audio books through an app on your phone. Yes ladies, it's time to be soothed as someone once again reads you that book at bedtime!

24.   Keep a 'phone handy

You will probably get lots of calls from friends and family to find out how you're doing after you get home from hospital, and one of the most frustrating things about having a hysterectomy is constantly getting up and down to answer the 'phone if you still have a landline.

Whilst it's good to exercise your abdominal muscles to help them heal, you also want to enjoy the recuperation time.

Your mobile phone should be kept close by, together with its charger. Make sure you check and change your data plan if necessary, if you plan to use it for more than a few texts or phone calls. You can also take it into hospital so you can provide updates to concerned friends and family.

When you decide to start the one-in-three challenge from our daily email hints and tips, don't forget to take your mobile with you; then, if you find you've overdone it at least you can call a 'taxi' to pick you up and take you home.

If you don't have, or don't want a mobile, why not change the landline to a hands-free set with three phones, that way you can keep the base set near the phone point and then have one upstairs and the other in the sitting room or kitchen.

But, remember this is your time to recover and you could really rebel and ignore the phone when it rings. Turn the volume down on your mobile and let calls go to the answer phone, and set up 1571 on your landline so that people can leave a message if your home phone doesn't have an answer phone. You can then get back to them later, if you really want to.

25.   Be calm and relaxed

If you're calm and relaxed prior to your operation, you'll need less anaesthetic, your muscle tone won't interfere with surgery, you will heal faster physically and your overall recovery time will be shorter.

Sounds good, you'll have some of that? So, how do you achieve it?

First, you've got to be sure in your own mind that a hysterectomy is right for you and that you're in control. If you still aren't sure, refer to hints 1, 10 and 11 and take any actions you need to.

Next, you need to be able to visualise in vivid detail how much better your life will be post recovery.

Divide one page of your journal in two. On one side of the page write about how much your health problems have held you back and affected your work, family, social life and relationships.

Now, on the other side write down how you will use the post-recovery benefits when released from those drawbacks.

The important thing in this exercise is to use detail. For example, what does pain look like, smell like, taste like? We experience the world through our senses but many in the west have lost the ability to recognise it. And, when you are describing the benefits, use the details to make it real for you, as if you're experiencing all those benefits now.

Finally, whenever you feel frightened, worried, are in pain, uncomfortable or just feeling down, revisit your list and relive the destinations that you set out on this journey to achieve, and give yourself a big pat on the back for getting this far.

When you combine this exercise with your journal entries and the scaling diary I talk about in the next section, this one of the most powerful ways to face and recover from, major surgery.

26.   Time to talk

The time before and after a hysterectomy can be disruptive for relationships of all kinds. From work, to children, your family and friends right through to your significant other; it can seem as if a slice of life has been removed.

Many women on the helpline describe how their work and leisure time has had to accommodate detailed planning on every single thing for a week or two each month, twelve times a year. Your mood may have swung all over the place; tears one minute, incandescent rage the next. And, your closest relationships have also had to cope with this too. Your hysterectomy may well be opening a whole new life and it's time to talk about what you want this to be like. The most important person to do this with is your partner, although you may want to have a similar conversation with other people you are close to as well.

Do you and your partner communicate well? Do they know of your hopes and fears about your hysterectomy? Do you know what about your surgery worries them?

A non-confrontational way of talking about how you view life after hysterectomy is to play a 'needs and expectations game', where you each write down what you believe the other person needs (can't do without) and expects (would like to have) after your hysterectomy are.

When you've written them down, swap your lists and use the insights gained as way of starting a conversation.

This can open a new world of possibility by removing previous blocks and misunderstandings. You can laugh at the assumptions you made about each other, cry at the things you are both worried about and be amazed where you find yourselves saying exactly the same thing.

Your closest relationships are the people you will turn to immediately after surgery, they will be the lynch pin your recovery time revolves around and this exercise will help you all feel as if you are moving in the same direction, together.

27.   Check your oestrogen levels for long term health

If you have a hysterectomy that removes your ovaries, your levels of oestrogen will drop quickly.

If you're past the menopause you need to be mindful that you may have a return of some menopausal symptoms. This is because we continue to produce lesser amounts of oestrogen long after our menopause has finished. The symptoms won't be as dramatic as they were, but are noticeable by many women.

If you haven't yet been through the menopause, it will start immediately and is called a surgical menopause.

If you are pre-menopausal and your ovaries are left in place, you still have a fifty percent chance of them failing within five years of surgery and so going into the menopause early.

If you are planning to keep your ovaries, it can be helpful to have your blood oestrogen levels measured before your hysterectomy takes place. This will give your GP something to compare future results against if you do experience unusual symptoms.

Oestrogen levels can be measured with a simple blood test, and several may be taken over the course of your cycle prior to surgery to get a good baseline result. Falling levels of oestrogen in your blood tests after your hysterectomy can be a good indicator that your ovaries are failing. This is the point at which you can decide about how to navigate through the menopause.

28.   Banish Superwoman syndrome

Most women think they're superwoman.

Not only may we have a job; we often take responsibility for the bulk of the shopping, cooking, cleaning, laundry and running the household. We get involved in outside activities, may be our family taxi and generally run ourselves ragged. We make sure everyone eats regularly, has done their homework and is wearing clean knickers (just in case they get run over).

The problem with a hysterectomy is the image we have of ourselves being superwoman takes a bit of a battering and about time too!

Let's face it, our partners are perfectly capable of cooking a meal, doing the grocery shopping, hanging washing out and doing the ironing; our problem is we think they don't do it right, so we must do it 'properly'.

Now is the time to let the standards slip a little and to accept with gracious thanks, all the efforts made by our families and friends that help make our recovery just that little bit easier.

If your partner doesn't know one end of a wash cycle from another, do a show and tell and then get them to do it; write out instructions beginning with sorting the laundry into the right piles.

If they don't know what to buy in the weekly shop, make it easy and give them a list of the things you buy every week; you never know some welcome treats might come home as well.

The advantage of all this preparation, of course, is that when you are back on your feet again, there can be no more excuses to avoid sharing the household tasks!

An even bigger bonus is that when your significant other understands that stacking the dishwasher, loading the washing machine and doing the ironing are not done by fairies, but is making a significant difference to your recovery, they might get more brownie points from you than they've had all day and that's got to be good for the relationship.

29.   Do I need progesterone?

Progesterone (progestin) is used by the female body to help maintain pregnancy, protect against the 'build-up' effect of oestrogen which is linked to womb and breast cancer and prevent ovulation taking place in the second half of the menstrual cycle.

After the menopause, the production of progesterone stops and if you have a hysterectomy that removes the ovaries then your progesterone production will stop as well. There is some research which suggests that progestins also have a positive influence on bone, heart, brain and other tissues, and that they may be beneficial for women that cannot take oestrogen[12]. However, other research suggests that higher levels of progesterone may be a risk factor in breast cancer[13].

If you feel that progesterone might be beneficial then it could be worth considering the herbal supplements Dong Quai and Black Cohosh as they are considered by complementary therapists to have similar effects. However, if you are having a hysterectomy because of cancer then you may be advised to avoid both of these alternative remedies because of their oestrogenic effects.

30.   Organise your child care

Do you still have young or school age children? If so, managing child care is more than just arranging for someone to pick them up from school or look after them in the holidays.

How about finding out about the local after-school clubs so your partner, parents or friends can collect them after work. And, why not talk to other parents about how to manage the school run, ask for help - the worst they can say is 'No'.

You will also need to think about the needs of very young children as you won't be able to pick them up for a few weeks, and they won't be able to jump on top of you.

Maybe some of the activities you always do together, such as swimming might need to stop or be done with someone else for a while. But, don't just stop them on the day you come out of hospital; it is important you explain to all your family what your hysterectomy will mean for you in terms of the things you can and can't do as you recover, and how it will affect them. Do this well before the day of the operation so they can prepare as well.

31.   Get your hair cut

Getting your hair cut can be a straightforward way of helping you feel better about yourself in the short term, while recovering from your operation. Not only will you look good, but getting it cut in a way that is easy to look after means you don't have to worry too much about hair gels, sprays and styling while recovering.

One thing you won't want to do for a few weeks is lift your arms up for long periods of time to hold a hairdryer and brush as this will pull on your traumatised tummy muscles.

Personally, I'd go for something young and funky; you won't look, or feel your years when you see yourself in the mirror.

To get the perfect haircut, book in a long appointment with your favourite stylist and talk over with them what suits the shape of your face and the image you would like. Take along a few pictures you've found in magazines of the styles you like for inspiration. Remember though, the need is for something simple to care for, not complicated or fussy.

One thing's for sure, you won't regret it afterwards and there does seem to be a strong anecdotal ink between looking good and feeling better.

32.   Give blood

For most women, their hysterectomy operation goes without a hitch. However, for the occasional few there may be problems, which could result in a serious loss of blood.

If you have an unusual blood type it may be worth discussing with your GP and/or gynaecologist whether it is possible to make a blood donation, specifically for use in the event of a problem. In the event your blood isn't needed by you, it could then be donated to the general blood bank.

As well as making a donation of blood, having a really good blood count is important for your long-term recovery and to help prevent anaemia. With this in mind, it is probably worth increasing your intake of green leafy vegetables and perhaps offal such as liver, which are a good source of iron.

Other sources of iron include: lamb, beef, soya, shell fish such as mussels, lentils, kidney beans, tofu, dried apricots, oatmeal (porridge), chickpeas, quinoa and blackstrap molasses. However, as iron from food sources isn't easily absorbed by the body, you may want to add a vitamin C rich foods to the same meals as this will help the take up of iron.

Vitamin C is often found in strongly pigmented foods such as carrots and peppers, oranges and apples.

When you've had your operation, it may be a good idea to ask for a blood count to be done (if they don't do one as a matter of course), just to check that your iron levels are up to scratch.

33.   Pet therapy

Research has shown that heart attack victims who have pets live longer. Apparently, even watching a tank full of tropical fish may lower blood pressure, at least temporarily.

It has long been known that pet ownership affects people positively both physiologically and psychologically, as the soothing, relaxing effect of stroking or sitting with a pet slows your heart rate down.

Pets are also wonderful to have around when you aren't feeling well as they often sense what you need and will be there for you; no need to talk, no need to explain, all you need to do, is 'be'.

The positives aside, if you have a pet you will need to think about the practicalities, especially if you live alone.

Will you book Harry into the local kennels or can a friend have Tom for you (apologies to those of you with a partner called Harry or Tom!)? Can you persuade a friend to pick up pet food on the weekly shop or order it online for delivery?

A dog walker or sitter could be booked in advance and be a fantastic investment after you get home from hospital; you won't have to worry about walking further than you're able to, or being pulled over.

34.   Buy a support cushion

After your hysterectomy, you will spend quite a lot of time sitting and reclining on a bed or chair, and a good support cushion can be a real investment.

These V shaped cushions, which are available from most bed linen stockists, help to keep your back, neck and shoulders well supported and can be used on chairs, sofa's and beds.

You could even take it into hospital with you for maximum comfort during your stay.

In the hospital

35.   Use a scaling diary

Half the battle in getting over a hysterectomy physically, mentally and spiritually is seeing an improvement each day in the things that are important to you. Your first task then, is to decide what you want to achieve and what's important to you.

For example, you might want to be able to walk a mile in the first three weeks (our one in three challenge); or, you might want to go out for coffee with friends during the second week at home; you might decide that getting back to work is your priority, or being able to do the hobbies you've set aside for a while.

Everyone is different so our goals are going to be different too. What's right for you, doesn't have to be right for anyone else, and vice versa.

When you've decided what's important, then you can think of the things that might influence whether you can, or can't do something. It might be that you need to have less pain, can walk longer, are able to get up and down the stairs easily or are less tired. Again, everyone is different and the way we recover is different too.

We've put together an example of the types of things you might want to monitor during your recovery and you can get started right now by thinking about the following, marking off where you feel you are right now.

At the end of this book is a page you can use as a template for your own scaling diary, or you can make your own up before you go into hospital.

Day: ..../ Date: .... / Time: ....
(1 is the least/lowest you've had or done and 10 is the most/highest you've had or done)

Pain	1	2	3	4	5	6	7	8	9	10
Sleeping	1	2	3	4	5	6	7	8	9	10
Mood	1	2	3	4	5	6	7	8	9	10
Tiredness	1	2	3	4	5	6	7	8	9	10
Exercise	1	2	3	4	5	6	7	8	9	10
Comments:										

For the first week or two you could fill it in two or three times a day, and this will help you see patterns emerge. Use this together with your hysterectomy recovery journal and, within a couple of weeks, you'll be able to see how much you're improving; small baby steps towards it at first, and then big giant leaps later on.

And don't forget contact *resources@hysterectomy-association.org.uk* to request your free set of resources to download that accompany this book, including some A4 scaling diary pages.

36.   Drink plenty of water, the greatest healer

Around fifty-five to sixty percent of our bodies are made up of water, in fact the brain is more than seventy percent water by weight and, if it dips below its critical level, you will feel listless, dull and very light headed. It is no wonder then that we need to drink a lot just to manage our daily lives.

After your hysterectomy, you will be dehydrated and your body will be trying to rid itself of toxins, such as the anaesthetics; you will also be at risk of developing a urinary tract infection because of any catheters that have been inserted.

However, by taking lots of liquids, especially plain water, you will be giving your body the best chance of avoiding any of these problems. As well as flushing the body out, it will also help to keep your stools soft, so that they are easier to pass and it will help you go to the loo regularly as well.

The recommended intake is around one and a half to two litres per day. This can be in plain water, weak teas, herbal and fruit teas, milk, fruit juice and squash and you can tell when you're drinking enough, because your urine will be pale in colour.

To make it easier to drink, why not take a sports water bottle into hospital with you and ask friends, relatives or the nurse to fill it regularly. That way you won't have to move about too much to take frequent drinks and don't risk spilling anything either. And if you don't like plain tap water, add a slice of lemon or lime to brighten it up a bit.

37. Relaxation and meditation

There is no doubt about it, being calm and relaxed before any type of surgery is the best approach; being stressed and fearful may increase the risk of any side effects or other problems during your hysterectomy or later recovery.

There are lots of different ways to achieve a calm mind before surgery and which you prefer will be as individual as you are. However clinical studies do show that several types of mindfulness exercise do have positive effects on stress which may include slowing the heart rate and even reducing blood pressure[14]. There are even studies to show that it helps reduce levels of pain, but more about that later.

One of the easiest ways to practice mindfulness is to use a guided meditation recording you download or play on a CD. Just remember not to do so when you're driving!

Listen to the guided meditation CD or download for a week or so before your hysterectomy, either before bedtime or at some other quiet point in the day when you won't be disturbed.

Once you get back from hospital, you can then use it whenever you feel the need to relax in the morning, afternoon and evening. It will help you maintain a relaxed state of mind while your body takes over the job of getting you fit and well again.

Don't forget to track when you use it in your journal so you can see the positive effects it's having on your own goals.

38.   Get your bowels moving

There are several reasons for a sluggish bowel post hysterectomy; anaesthetics used during surgery are designed to prevent muscle movement and as such it can take time for the bowel and bladder to 'wake up'.

Add to this dehydration and pain and you have the most common reasons why women have problems getting back into a regular bowel rhythm after a hysterectomy. All three can prevent the bowel from opening properly, particularly when the expectation of pain is high. In some hospitals, though, you won't be allowed to leave hospital until you have had at least one bowel movement.

Drinking lots of water and other weak fluids, as well as warm water and lemon juice first thing in the morning will help enormously. A gentle laxative or some natural fibre added to your breakfast cereal will probably deal with the most stubborn cases.

Once you're at home, gently massaging your abdomen in a clockwise direction, being careful not to rub too hard, will encourage the normal motion of the bowel; and by taking supplements such as fish and olive oils, you can help to keep the stools soft so that they don't become dry, hard and too painful to pass.

Of course, plenty of fibrous fruit and vegetables are a great addition to your diet and many women have begun increasing eating dietary fibres and drinking lots of water, a week or two before their operation.

Finally, lack of our usual level of exercise, even if it's just walking around the house, has a surprising effect on our ability to clear our bowels, so the sooner you can get out of bed and start moving physically again, the better.

39.   How do I get out of bed?

It's amazing how many of the abdominal muscles you use doing things we all take for granted such as getting out of bed. After a hysterectomy, it can become a real effort and takes a lot of thinking to achieve. The following suggestion seems to work for most women.

1. Shuffle over to within about twelve inches of the side of the bed you would like to get out of;
2. pull your knees up so your heels are against your bottom and slowly turn over on your side facing the edge of the bed;

3.   slowly, manoeuvre your knees and legs over the side of the bed and allow them to act as a counterweight as you push up with your arms until you are sitting upright on the side.

If you simply want to sit up in bed, pull your heels under your bottom and push hard into the mattress with your hands and feet to prevent using your abdominal muscles to pull you up. Incidentally this way of getting out of bed is also helpful if you ever suffer from a bad back!

40.   Affirmations for health

Having confidence in your own ability to help yourself heal is one of the keys to active wellness. Much of how well you feel is governed by your mood and attitude to life in general; if you expect things to go well and believe that you are going to be healthy and happy in the future, then the chances are that this is what you'll get.

To help get these positive feelings working for your benefit, you are going to devise your own affirmation.

It's important to remember, the key to affirmations is repetition; if you say them regularly and with conviction then you will retrain your subconscious mind to think in this new and positive way.

To get started, think about what you want to include; will it be no pain and freedom from the restrictions on your lifestyle, the new image you will have or the energy you can expect, or activities you can do?

Make your words and phrases fit with who you are, and make sure you keep it very much in the present. If you put it into the future then it will remain in the future.

You might say something like "I'm feeling full of energy and have no pain". At first it may feel a bit false, but the more you say it, the more you will feel it, so please do persevere.

When the affirmations are working to your satisfaction, you can change or expand them to include other things you want to change too.

As well as saying your own affirmations, why not ask your family and friends to keep you in their thoughts and send you a healing prayer or thought. Knowing that people are thinking of you and wishing you the very best, makes a positive statement about how much others value your presence in their life, and this makes you feel even better!

41.   Peppermint and other teas

One of the most uncomfortable side-effects of gynaecological surgery is wind, with many women rating it amongst the top three stressors.

It is a type of ileus and is caused by the manipulation of the bowel during abdominal surgery, creating additional gas which can be very painful to pass. Combined with a sluggish bowel due to the anaesthesia and you have a perfect storm of pain.

While a few hospitals now make peppermint tea or cordial available as a matter of course, unless yours is one of them; take your own. Not only is it good for wind, it's also good for the digestion, contains no caffeine, isn't a diuretic; and, when it's combined with honey, a natural sleep promoter.

And, it's not the only tea with therapeutic properties by a long chalk. Green Tea is a decongestant, anti-inflammatory, aids absorption of vitamins and boosts the immune system. Red Bush tea brightens you up, is low in caffeine and is a great for the digestive tract; while Siberian Ginseng tea restores immediate and long-term energy supplies, overcomes stress and fatigue and helps to maintain blood sugar levels. Finally, Oolong Tea is great for the digestion, is a natural stimulant and boosts positive mood.

42.   Help yourself prevent thrombosis

It is highly likely that before surgery you will be asked to put on some very sexy white surgical compression stockings.

These are put on before, or during, your hysterectomy to help prevent blood clots from forming in the deep veins of the legs during the operation and later, while you are spending much of your time in bed resting. DVT (deep vein thrombosis) is comparatively rare and affects around only one or two people in every 1000.

If you do get a DVT, then there are two possible complications that may occur; pulmonary embolus (a blood clot which travels to the lung), or post thrombotic syndrome (persistent calf symptoms). For these reasons, it is advisable to make sure that you do any exercises given to you by physiotherapy staff in the hospital.

You can also help to prevent any problems yourself by ensuring you drink plenty of water, which helps your circulation; and by walking as far as you can as soon after your hysterectomy as possible. The muscles in the lower legs act like little pumps and as you walk they help to keep the blood circulating and prevent it from forming clots.

Raising the level of your feet on pillows or cushions whenever you are resting will also take the pressure off your calf veins. The highest incidence of pulmonary embolus occurs within twenty-four hours after your hysterectomy, although they can happen up to three weeks later, so it is important to continue doing the exercises, walking, staying hydrated with plenty of water and keeping your legs raised during rest times, even when you get home.

43.   Managing pain

Pain is the body's way of telling us something is wrong and as we all know, it can range from simple discomfort to agony. Everyone feels it differently though as we don't have the same pain threshold.

After a hysterectomy, your pain will be managed in two ways. Initially, you will have a PCA (patient controlled analgesia) which has a needle inserted into the back of your hand usually, this normally contains morphine.

The advantage of a PCA device is that you can be in control of your pain medication. To deliver a shot, you simply press the button; a built-in timer stops you from overdosing. It is normally removed within the first twenty-four to forty-eight hours.

After your PCA device has been removed, you will be given regular painkillers such as paracetamol for surgical pain, depending on how much pain you are in.

Once you're at home, paracetamol will probably be advised, although you may feel you need something stronger, which your GP can prescribe. As you progress through your recovery, your need for pain control becomes less.

If, once you get home, you don't like the idea of taking too many tablets then you could consider combining them with a more natural approach, such as acupuncture or acupressure. Both operate on the principle of body 'trigger points' where applying a needle or finger pressure to a specific point will relieve pain. They can also stimulate the body to produce more endorphins (the body's natural pain relievers).

Visualising the natural healing process going on within your body is also very therapeutic, and it can help manage pain levels. Why not imagine you've packed the area in pain with ice, and gradually feel it freezing.

Don't forget to keep monitoring your levels of pain in your scaling diary. Not only will this show you how far you've come, but it can help you to spot any potential problems.

44. Make up a hospital basket

Let's face it, being in hospital is not going to be the most exciting time of your life and, although you will be meeting other women to talk to, you will probably want other things to do on the few days you're going to be in.

If you'd like a hand working out what to take into hospital, why not check out our hospital packing list, just search the Hysterectomy Association website.

Why not make up a basket of treats to take in with you containing a book, magazine, puzzle book, pens, notelets, don't forget to pre-load the apps on your phone with some meditations and audio books as well as your music.

Remember, the odd guided relaxation or meditation can work wonders to quell the nerves before your operation; and to help send you off to sleep after.

Don't forget your hysterectomy journal and scaling diary so you can monitor your progress from the start. And, what about including peppermint tea bags, mineral water and some fresh fruit juice to ensure you're drinking enough fluids.

Then there's the food. Fruit will give you an energy boost without overloading your system with refined sugars; dried fruit and nuts can help get your bowels moving and a piece of dark chocolate does give you a mental and emotional boost.

45.   Understanding what happens in hospital?

On *day one*, after your surgery, you will probably feel aches and pains all over your body, have a stiff-neck and abdominal pain (this can continue for several days).

You may find you are attached to patient controlled analgesia (PCA) device, do use it, you can't overdose.

You will almost certainly have a catheter inserted into your bladder so you don't have to worry about going to the loo to pass urine; at the same time, you will have a saline drip inserted into the needle in your arm to compensate for dehydration. Drink as much as possible, the more you drink, the sooner the drip will be removed.

Don't plan any visits except from your nearest and dearest as you will be drifting in and out of sleep and you don't want to feel responsible for maintaining a conversation.

On *day two*, your catheter will be removed if it hasn't already and you will be encouraged to get up and walk to the loo, with some support.

Once you're over the wobbles, try and walk as much as possible; don't go far, just around the bed or the ward at first, but the more you do, the better you will feel.

You may also have some discharge or slight bleeding, this is perfectly normal. The physiotherapists may come to show you some simple exercises to help prevent DVT, if they didn't do it before your operation.

Encourage any visitors to keep it brief and bring some lovely flowers.

If you have had a minimally invasive hysterectomy you may even be allowed to go home today as long as you can urinate and have had a poo.

On *day three*, have a warm and gentle shower, you'll feel so much better, but try and keep your dressing and the wound dry.

By now you should be thinking about opening your bowels, if this doesn't happen, then ask for a mild laxative and drink as much warm water as possible. Some hospitals will also ask for a blood test to be done to check you aren't anaemic.

You may find you feel quite low and weepy and once again this is perfectly normal.

Depending on the type of hysterectomy you had, and how well you are recovering, you may also be allowed to go home today.

Most women will be home on days three to five and, depending on the hospital policies, you will be able to join the escape committee and start your recovery proper at home.

When you're heading home, ask someone to bring in something loose and comfortable to wear for the drive home, you don't want tight waist bands digging into your tender tummy.

Don't forget your recovery pillow; tucked inside the seat belt will prevent any rubbing or chaffing or knocking.

These are the average times for most women, but your hospital may be different, so do make sure you collect any leaflets or information packs.

Recovery Time

46.   Create a relax corner

Taking care of yourself is your number one priority when you get home from hospital. And, making sure you don't have to get up and down too frequently by creating a cosy corner just for you is essential.

A comfortable chair or the end of the settee with lots of soft cushions and a big footstool, or low table piled with cushions, to put your feet up on will get you started. Add a side table and large box or basket handy for keeping books, magazines, phone, bottled water and a thermos of tea close to hand.

If you have a tablet, MP3 player or are using a mobile phone, make sure there's a handy socket for their power adapters and, if necessary, buy an extension lead long enough to reach your corner. Add remote controls for things like the stereo and TV. If you are using CD's for healing relaxation and meditation then don't forget to stack them handily with your CD player.

Finally, your recovery cushion, a warm blanket and hot water bottle If you feel the cold will complement your cosy corner, keeping everything within arm's reach, so you only have to get up to do your regular walks, go to the loo or fill the thermos flask.

Don't forget to let everyone in the house know that this is your special, personal space to be used only by you while you're recovering.

And, if you are lucky enough to be recovering over the summer when the weather is good, why not create it in a nice shady nook in the garden, if you have one, for the day.

47.   Inner cleansing drink

Pineapple is high in the enzyme bromelain which is a natural anti-inflammatory that also encourages healing. Limes are full of vitamin C, as is apple juice and they are both full of anti-oxidants.

- ❖   1 carton live yoghurt
- ❖   1 small can unsweetened pineapple chunks
- ❖   1 small bottle of freshly pressed apple juice
- ❖   Juice of 1 lime
- ❖   Drizzle of honey to taste (if required)
- ❖   Handful of ice to cool it all down

Pop all the ingredients in a blender and blend into a really thick, smooth drink. Decorate with a slice of lime, if you fancy, and sip it over the course of an hour.

48. Pelvic floor exercises

The pelvic floor muscles are two groups of muscles situated around the urethra, vagina and anus. They provide support to your womb, bladder and bowel.

After your womb is removed, the other organs will shift around the abdomen and you now have a slightly increased risk of prolapse of these organs later in life.

Pelvic floor exercises (Kegel exercises) help to stabilise your inner core muscles, providing strength and support, and are useful to help prevent prolapse and urinary incontinence. They also tone up the vagina as well.

To do them effectively you need to alternately contract and relax the pubococcygeus muscle, which is the one that controls your urine flow. The simplest way to do the exercise is to locate the muscle by trying to stop the flow of urine the next time you go to the loo.

Once you have identified where the muscle is and what it feels like to contract it you can do the following exercise whenever and wherever you want to.

Pull the muscles up for a count of five and then relax. Repeat this process ten times, two or three times daily.

49.   The value of walking

One of the easiest ways to get the exercise you need after your hysterectomy is to walk. Walking helps improve your circulation, gets the bowel moving and guards against deep vein thrombosis.

It calms your mind, helps you relax and just thirty minutes a day of brisk walking when you are fully recovered will mean your heart remains healthy, as well as keeping the weight off.

You will almost certainly be encouraged to get out of bed the day after surgery, or even before if your surgery was early in the morning; this is your cue to start your walking regime, increasing the distance a little each time.

At first, you can begin with walking around your bed, to the loo and back or even around the ward. As you feel more confident, why not venture out a short way along the hospital corridors. The trick is not to go so far you can't get back again. If you are worried about getting stranded, take a friend or relative along with you.

Your body will almost certainly want to hunch forwards to protect your abdomen, however, it will be better for your back if you try and walk upright; to help this why not buy an abdominal support band, they are designed specifically for this area of the body.

Don't forget to keep a note in your journal of how far you walk every day; every step around the ward or house counts too.

An exercise monitor such as a Fitbit, an app on your phone or even a simple pedometer will help you keep track of your walking progress; it will probably be further than you think.

50.   Get rid of water retention

Even the most unfit people exercise every day. Activities such as walking, going up and down stairs, household chores and shopping provide your body with a regular routine.

When you have a hysterectomy, this routine is disrupted and, because you aren't doing as much as usual, water retention can be common.

It can also be a side effect of some types of hormone replacement therapy. It appears as swelling in the ankles and lower legs or in the tummy area, some women may also experience it in their hands and fingers; and it can be very uncomfortable, as well as making you feel very self-conscious. In some cases, it can be so bad that you have problems putting shoes on or rings on your fingers.

Despite your natural inclination not to drink too much, increasing your water intake to around one and half to two litres a day can help as it means your body isn't holding onto fluids because it feels dehydrated.

As well as increasing the amount of water you drink, limiting the amount of salt you eat and increasing the distances and frequency of walking are all beneficial; walking helps because the muscles at the bottom of the legs act a little like pumps that get blood and lymph fluids circulating.

Increasingly, medical studies are showing that sitting for long periods of time is as unhealthy for us as doing no exercise at all, so a short walk every hour that builds distance gradually may be more effective than one long walk each day.

Dandelion and parsley supplements are both natural diuretics and you could also try drinking fennel tea. Adding fennel oil to a warm bath will have a similar effect or why not massage your body, particularly your legs, with fennel diluted in carrier oil?

51.   Aloe Vera juice and Cat's Claw

Around 3000 years ago, seriously wounded Roman soldiers were sent to an island colonised by plants with spiky, rubbery leaves. They found that by drinking the juice and by rubbing a freshly broken leaf on a wound, they healed twice as quickly as their colleagues.

Nowadays, we also appreciate the many other virtues of one of nature's most powerful healers, both internal and external. Many people keep a plant around the house as an emergency first aid kit, breaking a small part off a leaf and rubbing it on the affected area when they burn themselves

Many conditions are reputed to respond to Aloe Vera juice including candida, chronic fatigue, low immune system, ulcers, viral infections, arthritis, colds and digestive tract problems including irritable bowel syndrome.

Externally, Aloe Vera preparations are available to ease aches and pains and it also helps sunburned skin (if you were planning a holiday before or after your surgery).

Cat's Claw - Uncaria tormentosa - (so named for its appearance) is possibly one of the world's most important herbal discoveries. From the Peruvian rain forest, this herb works at many levels within the body, its reported therapeutic benefits[14] are linked to candida and cancer, allergies, intestinal disorders, depression and HIV.

Apparently, when Cat's Claw is used in conjunction with Aloe Vera, the effects can be profound. Both impact positively on the immune system and have been shown to have anti-viral, anti-inflammatory and antioxidant properties, acting like an immune stimulator.

As with all complementary therapies, check their use with your GP beforehand, especially if you are taking other medication, and do make sure you follow the manufacturer's instructions.

52.   Flower power relaxation exercise

The sight and smell of flowers is very uplifting and their scent can be very heady causing an emotional response in us that encourages our body to release 'feel good' hormones.

As well as being given flowers, you can also imagine them in this simple relaxation exercise.

Settle down somewhere comfortable with your feet raised and your back supported;

Breathe deeply for five breaths;

Close your eyes and breathe in through the nose and out through the mouth;

Allow your inner vision to show you a beautiful bud;

It slowly unfurls, petal by petal, imagine each petal opening contributing to a beautiful flower in full bloom;

Watch the flower in your mind's eye, mentally turn it so you can see it from different angles and relax;

Remember, that this is what you are, a flower that is slowly unfurling its petals and coming into full bloom.

The flowers you choose for your relaxation exercise also have potent meanings, for instance the Azalea is the Chinese symbol of womanhood and the chrysanthemum means cheerfulness, optimism, rest and truth. The Daffodil is associated with re-birth and new beginnings and Yarrow is for healing.

If you'd like to know the meaning of your favourite flower why not have a look at the following website: *www.almanac.com/content/flower-meanings-language-flowers.*

53.   Choose comfy, loose clothes

When you first come home from hospital, stay in your nightwear as much as possible for at least a week. Not only will this be one less thing to worry about, it will also help other people remember you are recovering from a major operation, and therefore not to expect too much from you. If you are walking, you can either stay local in the house and garden, or get dressed only when you need to, getting back into your nightwear as soon as you get home.

You'll know when you want to be up and dressed every day, especially as you increase the distance of your walks as there's no guessing about what could happen if you go out in just your new nighty!

Loose clothes, such as princess line dresses that fall from just below the bust, sports style tops and bottoms and loose elasticated and drawstring skirts and trousers, whilst not the most fashionable of items, will keep your tummy area free of restriction and, if you do have any wounds, prevent anything from chaffing on them.

Loose and full tops worn over what's on the bottom help disguise the elastic and cord ties. T-shirts and tops in bright colours also distract other peoples' eyes from your bottom half and have the added benefit of cheering you up as well.

Try to avoid tights and other close-fitting underwear, and stick to socks when you need to put something on your feet.

54.   Relieve shoulder tension and pain

When we are in pain or anxious we may hold parts of our body in uncomfortable ways. One of the most common is to hunch the shoulders up around the ears; in fact, why not do a reality check of your shoulders right now.

If they have floated up around your ears, bring them back down and relax your neck and jaw. You may notice that they ache when you bring them down, this is because they've got so used to being under tension, it feels 'wrong' for them to be in the right place.

This simple exercise will help keep your shoulders nice and supple and you can do it right after surgery, then carry on doing them for as long as you need when you get home. It's okay to do these sitting on a kitchen chair, one that allows you to hang your arms straight down by your sides.

- ❖ Sit or stand up straight, try to get your head balanced nicely at the top of your spine with your eyes facing forwards;
- ❖ Let your arms hang straight naturally by your sides and feel the weight of the hands pulling them down;

❖ Push your shoulders down as far as they will go and then lift them up to your ears and roll them back down again. Do this ten times;

❖ Now reverse the direction you rolled your shoulders, if you were rolling them backwards before, roll them forwards now; do this ten times.

You might notice crackling noises as you do the exercise and it might also cause a little pain when you start, don't worry it's just your body telling you that your shoulders need to release.

55. Grab some helpful supplements

There is no doubt about it, having surgery is a testing time for your body and some extra help would be very much appreciated.

Whilst there are lots of vitamins and minerals you could take, the following are a small selection that have an immediate effect on health after surgery.

For instance, vitamin C is used by the body for tissue repair and growth as well as for healing wounds, but the body can't retain it and so it needs to be replenished daily. It also needs zinc to be absorbed properly, so supplements with both together are better than a single variety of vitamin C.

Zinc is one of the most important trace minerals for our bodies as it has a major part to play in maintenance of body tissue and our immune system. It is also called the 'healing mineral' as it speeds up the healing process.

Vitamin E promotes the production of new blood cells and selenium is a key antioxidant that works in combination with vitamin E to protect our cells from free radicals and improve immunity; it is also an anti-inflammatory and believed to help with menopausal symptoms.

Perhaps the easiest way to take any of these healing helpers is in a good quality multi-vitamin and mineral supplement.

And don't forget to check with your GP that there will be no adverse reactions to any other drugs you're taking.

56.   Make a healing smoothie

If you don't fancy taking tablets, why not try our recipe for a healing smoothie; it's tasty and full of vitamin C, vitamin E and selenium as well as others your body will love to have.

❖ 1 small bottle/cup of freshly squeezed orange juice
❖ Handful of strawberries (fresh or frozen)
❖ Large teaspoon of wheat germ

Whizz all the ingredients together in the blender and pour into a large glass, decorate with fresh mint, if you feel like it. Then sit down, relax and enjoy the moment.

57. Perfect relaxation

Entering a more relaxed state will help to calm any physical tension so you are able to respond to creative, healing and positive thoughts.

The first thing to think about is how do you normally relax? Some people can get lost in music, others achieve inner peace in a garden, while yet more may be in a world of their own when dancing or reading. Whilst anyone can listen to music, whatever their state of health; it won't be so easy to dance or garden until you have recovered.

One effortless way of relaxing is by using visualisation; try this one out for size and adapt it to suit.

1. Make yourself comfortable and cosy somewhere you won't be disturbed for thirty minutes or so.

2. Think of a place or time when you were happy and relaxed. It might have been on a beach or in a wood; it could be a perfect afternoon in the garden, or that night on the dance floor when free expression and the music took over. Whatever you choose, you need to be able to recreate it vividly in your mind's eye.

3. Close your eyes. Become aware of your breathing, consciously taking slightly longer to breathe out.

4. Empty your mind of all your day to day concerns and go back to that special time and place.

5. Play it back to yourself.

6. Recall the sounds, smells, temperature, people and feelings.

7. Stay in the moment for as long as possible and enjoy the happy feelings to the full; feel good about yourself, smile inside and feel the love.

8. When you're ready, open your eyes and come back to the world around you.

While you were away in your imagination, your breathing and heart will have slowed down; your brain was releasing pleasure hormones and your immune system was being pumped up with energy and your muscles were relaxing.

Now you're back; how do you feel? You can repeat this exercise as frequently as you need to.

Don't forget to write down in your journal anything you remember about your special time, any effects felt after relaxing and anything else that feels important.

58. Ten things you shouldn't do for four to six weeks

- ❖ No vacuuming
- ❖ No lifting (anything more than a half full kettle)
- ❖ No sex (until the top of your vagina has healed)
- ❖ No driving
- ❖ No bending, unless you use your knees and keep your back straight

❖ No stretching to get things off a high shelf or hanging washing out

❖ No bed making

❖ No gardening

❖ No stacking or unstacking the dishwasher and washing machine unless you get down on your knees to do so

❖ Definitely no skateboarding!

In our resources pack are some pages with a list which you can photocopy and put on a convenient cupboard or wall to tell the whole family what you can, and CAN'T do, while you are recovering.

If you request our resources to download you'll find an A4 copy of the list to print out instead. Just email *resources@hysterectomy-association.org.uk* for more information.

59.   The joy of massage

Massage is one of the nicest ways to help your body heal itself, while giving yourself a good pampering at the same time. You don't necessarily have to go to a professional as it is possible to self-massage, particularly for bloating, dispelling wind and general relaxation.

The kneading, pummelling, stroking and rubbing of massage relieves muscle tension and triggers the release of endorphins. At the same time, most forms of massage also act on the lymphatic system, helping to remove toxins from the body. Because of this, you must remember to drink more water than usual after a massage to help the body flush those toxins away.

When you're ready to think about having sex with your partner again, massage can be one way of easing you both into it by helping to relax the muscles that you might tense in anticipation of experiencing the same pain you may have had before your hysterectomy.

And, aromatherapy massage can be beneficial for managing the pain of any urinary tract infections you may have, particularly by massaging rosemary oil diluted in a carrier oil into your legs. If you find yourself suffering from water retention, then a lower back and abdominal massage, by your partner, with carrier oil and either grapefruit, carrot seed or juniper oil may help to ease the discomfort.

Why not try this simple hand massage while you're home alone.

1. Squirt a few drops of your favourite hand cream in to the palm of one hand;
2. Use your thumb to rub the cream into the heal of each hand using a firm circular motion;
3. Next, massage the web of skin between your thumb and forefinger, using a strong pulling motion;
4. Massage the base of the finger joints firmly;
5. Finally, lace the fingers together and massage the palms of each hand with your thumb.

60.   Relaxing reflexology

Reflexology is a wonderful technique as it uses nothing more than strategically placed finger pressure to relieve stress and other health problems. Reflexologists say the technique relieves tension, improves circulation and enhances nerve function.

The heel area of your feet relates to the pelvic area and the points around the outside of the ankle are associated with the female reproductive organs in particular. Gentle massage of this area could help to stimulate the body's natural healing processes, but be careful as it might be quite painful to touch too firmly.

Another useful reflexology point to know about is the base at the web of skin between the thumb and forefinger, which when gently rubbed can help to ease a tension headache.

61.   A little live yoghurt goes a long way

After any major surgery, your body is going to be in crisis, and finding ways to overcome this is the key to getting back on your feet as quickly as possible.

One way of supporting your system, after a diet of anaesthetics, pain killers and antibiotics, is by taking live yoghurt daily.

Lactobacillus acidophilus, which is one of the main constituents of live yoghurt, has been found to have a positive effect in maintaining, or regaining, the body's natural pH level as well as increasing our body's levels of 'good' bacteria[15].

Of course, when choosing your brand of live yoghurt, make sure you get a natural one rather than the flavoured or fruit ones, as the additional sugars included in them could undo some of the benefits you could see.

62. Invest in a few chick flicks

Once you get out of hospital you're not going to be able to do very much, so why not take the opportunity to borrow, rent, or buy, all those films you've said you wanted to watch in the past.

Nothing too stressful mind, because you won't want to tense your tummy muscles too much, but a little laughter (with your handy recovery cushion to hand) could be just what the doctor ordered.

If you have a DVD player, your friends and family could loan you theirs, or join the local library as they often have selection of DVD's and talking books. You could ask your partner, a friend or relative to change them for you when you can't get there for yourself.

Alternatively, you could join one of the video streaming services such as NetFlix, Sky Movies or Amazon Prime, that way you have access to both TV boxed sets as well as the latest films.

And, if you think you might have a problem expressing any emotions that come up after your hysterectomy, then an old fashioned weepy is a good excuse to cry without needing to offer any explanations to anyone else.

63.   Simple abundance

It is easy when we're recovering from a major operation to forget to be thankful for everything that is going right in our lives. From living in the UK where we can access medical care reasonably easily, free of charge (most of the time), and where many of us can take time off from our daily lives to get on with the task of getting better. Just spending time 'being' is one of the most important things you can do to aid your recovery. And appreciating all the little 'gifts' that come your way can be very therapeutic.

In your journal why not keep a Simple Abundance record as well, by listing four or five things about the day that were good and that you really appreciated.

It might be as simple as being able to sit in the garden for the afternoon with your book, having your partner do all the laundry, a visit from family and friends, or someone doing the shopping for you. Often it will be things you don't get the time to enjoy very frequently, because normal life gets in the way that makes these little things seem much more special.

It doesn't have to be much, but it's surprising how concentrating on the good things, make the bad seem less significant somehow.

64.   Managing painful wind

There is no doubt that wind is going to be one of the most painful aspects of your recovery. You can feel the pain in different areas, the most common are the lower abdomen and the shoulders.

The reason it happens is due to two things; firstly, the bowel is manipulated to get it out of the way and any opening in the abdomen, even for minimally invasive surgery, introduces additional air into a sealed cavity; secondly, the anaesthetic shuts your normal bowel movements down as well, and it takes time for it to re-establish a normal pattern.

Fortunately, there are several tried and tested methods for getting rid of the pain, just pick the ones that appeals most to you.

❖   Drink peppermint tea or cordial
❖   Gently rub your tummy in a clockwise direction
❖   Take charcoal tablets
❖   Drink slightly gassy mineral or soda water
❖   Chew chewing gum
❖   Walk

65.   Award yourself recovery treats

Why not think about rewarding yourself every time you do something different to help your recovery?

Let's say you walk a little more than your set distance for the day (without pain as you don't want to push yourself too hard just to get the treat), or drink a cup more than your daily amount of water, you could give yourself a treat?

Treats might include making a fresh fruit smoothie, visiting a friend, going out for coffee, buying some flowers or even indulging in a lovely long bath, after any wounds you have are fully healed.

To begin, make a list of all your Favourite Things (Oh yes, I forgot - singing like Julie Andrews!) so you have something to choose from without thinking too hard. When you decide you deserve it, choose the reward that gives you most pleasure.

With each reward tell yourself how much you deserve it, you're special and you're doing the very best that you can for your recovery right now.

66. Give a tender tummy support

After your hysterectomy, you naturally want to avoid activities that could actually help your tummy muscles recover. Deep breathing, coughing, laughing and walking upright can all seem a bit daunting because you expect to feel pain, and may worry you will damage any internal stitching.

It's normal to hunch forward every time you try anything involving the abdominal muscles, but it is important to straighten up. Good posture promotes healing by creating just enough tension in the abdominal muscles to strengthen them, without hurting your wound.

Bending forward to protect yourself, on the other hand forces you to lose your balance, discourages you from breathing deeply and can put additional strain on your back. You can hold your recovery pillow over your abdomen to help to keep the muscles firm when you laugh or cough; but there is a limit to how much you may want to take Cushion out with you when taking your daily walk!

When you get home after surgery you might find an abdominal support band helpful; they are designed to give gentle support to the whole abdominal region and your back, while you get your confidence back.

67.   Acupressure for constipation, diarrhoea and pain

Acupressure is a little like reflexology, in that parts of the body correspond with others and gentle pressure applied in those areas can relieve discomfort in the related area.

There are lots of acupressure points you could use to relieve all sorts of problems following surgery, but points on and around the hand are often easiest for you to use yourself.

❖   The first point is on the back of your hand, in the webbing between your index finger and thumb.

❖ Use your other thumb to locate the tender spot and apply gentle pressure deeply enough with your so you feel an achy or electrical sensation for a couple of minutes if you can bear it;

❖ Breathe in slowly and deeply while you are pressing.

Stimulating this point improves over all intestinal function and helps relieve constipation, diarrhoea and abdominal pain.

68.   Balancing hormones naturally

Our bodies need hormones to help regulate their normal functions and, if you have a hysterectomy that removes your ovaries, the most important ones to consider are oestrogen, testosterone and progesterone.

You may have decided that you don't want to, or can't, take hormone replacement therapy and will be thinking about what natural alternatives there may be available.

The menopause is an entirely natural cycle of life that all women will go through and there are now many natural remedies available in high street shops which are helpful for troublesome night sweats and hot flushes.

Some of the most important to look out for are those that contain phyto-oestrogens, these plant-based oestrogens are similar but less potent forms of the oestrogen we produce ourselves. You can find them a wide variety of foods such as Soya and Linseeds or even change your regular loaf for Burgen bread from your local supermarket. You'll also find a lot more information on the hysterectomy association website about complimentary approaches to dealing with menopausal symptoms.

If you are a baker then what about making your very own menopause cake, there's a recipe further along in the book that you can adapt to suit your own tastes.

However, as with HRT, you may find that it takes a while and a few false starts, before finding the best combination of supplements and diet for you. Don't give up and keep on trying. If you would like more information about how to manage the menopause naturally, then *'The New Alternatives to HRT'* by Marilyn Glenville is just about the best book available.

69.   Bach flower remedies

Dr Edward Bach devised thirty-eight homoeopathically prepared plant and flower based remedies to treat a variety of feelings and emotions. The most familiar to many people is Rescue Remedy, which is used to treat shock, including shock to the physical body (so it might be useful to take a bottle into hospital with you).

However, there are several others which can help support you physically and emotionally after having a hysterectomy.

Mimulus treats the fear of known things, such as fear relating to the operation itself or of not being able to cope afterwards.

Star of Bethlehem could help you deal with the after effects of shock.

Oak is good for those who are exhausted but are struggling to carry on, does that sound familiar for the superwoman in us?

Gorse is a great support if you have overwhelming despondency and despair.

Olive is helps the body manage a lack of energy, which is a common symptom after any type of surgery.

And finally, when you do have to face going back to work, use Hornbeam; it's good for that 'Monday morning feeling'.

70.   Am I still a woman?

Our body image is a key part of how we see ourselves in the world. Some women feel their essential essence is in being a mother and a few will feel that removal of their womb profoundly affects who they are and how others see them. Many other women don't have such an attachment to their female 'bit's but can still be surprised by strong reactions after they have a hysterectomy.

There is no right or wrong way to feel, as each is as valid and real as the other. Asking this question of yourself before your hysterectomy will help if you do experience a strong reaction or sense of loss; and can help begin the process of establishing a new understanding of your womanhood.

One woman I've spoken to has said that she coped by realising that the surgery had simply removed the nursery but left the playpen! This type of coping strategy is common amongst women who have children and feel their family is complete. For those of us who don't fall into this category our feelings may be very different.

We each need to ask ourselves what it is that makes us uniquely feminine. Writing these thoughts and emotions down in your hysterectomy journal allows you to process the feelings that could trip you up and then work out how to deal with them.

The reality of course is that you are still, and always will be, a woman, whether you have had a hysterectomy or not.

If you are troubled by your feelings after your hysterectomy, then you may find my book '*Losing the Woman Within*' very helpful. Part story, part information it is written by someone who has been there and experienced the full range of emotions after her hysterectomy.

71.   Listen to your body

You are the expert on your body and tuning into your own internal guidance system is a skill worth cultivating.

Your body is healthy in its natural state. Provide it with enough sleep, a good diet, exercise and plenty of water and it will respond by giving you the energy you need to live every day to the full.

However, now you've had a hysterectomy your body needs to let you know how best to help it back to health. And it's here that, providing you listen to your body, pain can be a positive asset in the healing process.

For the first few weeks after your operation, mark in your scaling diary the levels of pain you are feeling and at what times of the day and what you were doing/eating/drinking when it happened. Over time you'll see patterns emerge indicating what causes a problem and what works well. Doing more of the latter and less of the former will see you fit, healthy and whole in extra fast time.

72.   Bleeding and discharge

Many women are concerned when they get an unexpected bleed or discharge a few weeks after having a hysterectomy.

However, it is perfectly normal and can last from several days to several weeks. It usually becomes darker and turns into spotting as time goes on, but it can also be bright red. It's also common to experience some sort of vaginal discharge for a number of weeks.

Most post-operative bleeding is due to the normal healing process, the vagina expelling any clotted blood that has built up, or the stitches dissolving (this depends on the type of stitches used and how fast they dissolve).

Occasionally though, it can indicate you have overdone it, particularly if you've been doing a lot of heavier lifting, bending or stretching and usually, you would be able to pinpoint if this were the case.

The key with both bleeding and discharge is to see your GP if you are concerned, they continue for longer than six to eight weeks, if they change significantly, or are accompanied by other symptoms such as pain or fever.

73.　Slow down, and appreciate the day

How are you going to fix it so you take things easy for the first couple of weeks?

I've already talked about trying to be superwoman before the operation; now, what about being super-relaxed after?

Relaxation is the opposite of stress, and as stress can have a negative impact on your body, relaxation can be positive and healing. Stress and worry will ensure you don't heal as quickly as you could; relaxation and enjoying the moment will. The trick is understanding in advance what is likely to increase your stress levels.

Use your journal to note down what you think will really get on your nerves if it's not done? It may be housework such as bed making or cleaning the bathroom; gardening or related to your job.

Whatever it is you must find a way to get around it before you go into hospital. Would family and friends help? Or you could buy in the services of a cleaning company or gardener.

If your stress could be work related, think about what can you do before you go on sick leave to help colleagues who'll be covering for you? Perhaps, you could put together an instruction manual or do some coaching.

How tired you feel after your hysterectomy will be surprising, and taking the time to do nothing is one of the best gifts you can give yourself. You will be up and about and feeling fitter, much sooner than if you try to push yourself too early. So, give yourself a break and make getting better the most important 'job' you can do right now.

74.   Side effects of hysterectomy

There are many possible symptoms to experience after a hysterectomy; and you may have many or none. I've listed the most commonly reported so you can be aware of what is, and isn't, normal.

Most women say it takes up to six months before they are no longer thinking about having had a hysterectomy daily, and many will say it takes one to two years to fully recover.

❖   Incredible tiredness, can last several months, increasing your activity levels helps.

❖ Frequent and urgent need to go to the loo could indicate infection or irritation by the catheter.

❖ Pain around any wounds you have, this can be localised as well.

❖ Discharge or weeping around any wounds in the first week or two.

❖ Itching or burning around any wounds.

❖ Lack or sensation or numbness on one or both sides of the groin or legs, this eases over the first few weeks.

❖ Swelling around any wounds.

❖ Bloating and wind.

❖ Constipation or diarrhoea (especially if you had antibiotics).

❖ Vaginal discharge and/or smell (both may require some sort of antibiotic).

❖ Burning or itching around the vulva (this is often dryness and not yeast infection).

❖ Pain and swelling or redness at the site of intravenous needles.

❖ Pelvic cramps, which may be related to increased physical activity.

If you experience any of the symptoms above make sure you pay attention, use your journal if necessary. Anything that worsens or doesn't improve in a day or two should be reported to your GP.

75.   Look after your wounds

Around half of you will have a wound of some description after a hysterectomy, for most this will be a large incision either horizontal on the bikini line, or vertical from breast bone to below the naval. The rest will be small incisions on either side of the belly button that are used in more minimally invasive options.

It is important to take care of these wounds until they are all completely healed, this begins almost immediately and you can encourage it by keeping it (and any dressings) clean and dry until there is no discharge and the dressings come away dry when they are changed.

You could see some discharge coming from the wounds and although this could well be a normal part of your healing process. If you do get an infection then you will probably be prescribed some antibiotics or an antiseptic cream to use as directed by your GP.

After your wound has healed, rubbing Calendula cream or BioOil into the scar will help the skin to remain supple and prevent puckering.

Following immediate healing, your scar and the skin around it will be fragile for several months and most surgeons will recommend you avoid direct sunlight on the newly formed scar tissue. So, there'll be no flashing it around on the beach in Marbella this year.

76.   Write a poem to your womb

There is every chance that your hysterectomy will be a liberating experience. It could end years of symptoms that have been painful and difficult to live with, and give you opportunities to do things you couldn't before. It may even end uncertainty over your long-term health. These benefits though could mask an emotional upheaval as well.

A necessary part of the recovery process is coming to terms with a worry or symptoms which have dominated your life over previous months or even years. You may also experience a type of grief, that shows itself as shock, anger and resentment about how you have been affected by your problems and surgery; later this grief will adjust, allowing you to become hopeful for the future. The extent to which you feel these emotions will depend on many factors and there is no 'average' unfortunately.

Although it may seem a little left field or wacky, writing a poem to your womb, or your body in general, can give you an outlet for expressing the feelings you have held inside. Once these are out in the open you will be free to move on.

Pick up a pen and your journal and start writing down how you feel. Tell your body how much you have resented the problems it has caused, thank it for any children you have given birth to and finally tell it about how much you are going to enjoy your bright future.

77. Try some aromatherapy

Aromatherapy is a truly holistic therapy that takes the whole person into account. It acts on many senses at once and can be used to induce both healing and relaxation.

You can use the oils in many ways, but under no circumstances should you drink them. Instead put them into oil burners to benefit from the aroma, add small quantities to your bath water (but do remember to keep any wounds and dressings dry), dilute them with carrier oil and massage them into your skin, oil or add a few drops into a compress.

Those that might be most beneficial after a hysterectomy include some with antibacterial properties such as Tea Tree, Lavender, Eucalyptus, Bergamot and Juniper.

Jasmine, Bergamot, Geranium, Lavender and Ylang Ylang can all lift your mood and, if you would like to give your sex life a boost, then Ylang Ylang, Rose and Neroli are the ones to go for. Geranium also balances hormones, whilst Clary Sage, Fennel, Star Anise and Tarragon have some oestrogenic qualities which may be useful for managing menopausal symptoms.

78. Healing laughter

Laughing out loud beats almost any pill or potion as it releases a surge of 'feel good' hormones. The rush of energy it creates reduces fatigue and tension, slashes the production of stress hormones, boosts the immune system and protects the heart.

Think about how you rate on the laughter stakes; When was the last time you had a good belly-laugh? What makes you laugh? Are you a naturally humorous person? How many times a day do you laugh, or even smile.

When you've put all that in the balance consider whether you need a GSOH makeover; it really will help your recovery.

Make a list of the top ten things that get you chuckling, be they books, comics, films, TV box sets, magazines or your private hoard of recollections. Don't leave this handy hint until you've made the list, just add to it as another one springs to mind; once you've experienced the effects, you'll want to include laughter as an essential part of your daily recovery diet.

There is a health warning though, it can be painful in those early days after your hysterectomy, so put your recovery cushion over your tummy and wrap your arms around it to hold your muscles firmly.

79.   Understanding phytoestrogens

Phytoestrogens are chemicals of plant origin that mimic the action of the female hormone, oestrogen. Research suggests they can be helpful in reducing the severity of some menopausal symptoms[16], such as hot flushes and night sweats.

By supplementing the diet of some volunteers with soya beans, red clover and linseed oil, researchers found that the women's levels of FSH (Follicle Stimulating Hormone) which increases after the menopause, reduced to pre-menopausal levels. This could explain why Japanese women who have diets high in soya, are less likely to have any menopausal symptoms.

Other sources of phytoestrogens include whole grains, chickpeas, lentils, garlic, celery, rhubarb, alfalfa sprouts and parsley.

Perhaps the easiest way to take phytoestrogens is by increasing the amount of soya you eat. You could do this by adding soya yoghurt and milk to your diet, or even by substituting some of your usual flour for soya flour when, and if, you bake. However, make sure you go for the organic varieties as soya crops are amongst the most genetically modified. Your local health food store also probably stocks many supplements containing red clover and linseed.

80.   Get some R'n'R

R'n'R, rest and recuperation to you and me, is hard for many women as they take their responsibilities very seriously; but rest you must if you want to recover as quickly and easily as possible.

There are many different types of rest but one of the most important is bed rest, and in particular, sleeping.

Research shows that the body repairs and regenerates tissues, builds bone and muscles and appears to strengthen the immune system during non-REM (dreamless) sleep. Whilst REM (dreaming) sleep acts as a psychological safety valve, helping us work through unconscious events and emotional issues.

In addition to sleeping, being in bed and lying down means you aren't straining your abdominal muscles around the surgery site. It also relaxes your spine, allowing it to return to its natural posture. And, if you had your cervix removed, the vaginal area also needs time to heal without having the pressure of the remaining abdominal organs bearing down on it.

The key ladies, is to rest in bed as much as you can, for as long as you can. When you get bored or your body tells you it needs to move, get up and get moving by fitting in your daily walks. You can then potter back to bed for a few hours of helpful, restorative sleep.

81. Spread a little honey

Honey has long been thought to have many positive healing qualities, and in recent years it has been enjoying something of a revival in hospital wound care for skin abscesses. It acts as an antibacterial and antifungal agent and helps to disinfect the skin and speed up the healing process[17].

It has many unique nutritional and health benefits, too many to be listed here, although researchers in California have now shown that eating honey can also raise the levels of anti-oxidants in the body in the form of polyphenols that are thought to reduce the risk of heart disease and cancer. Polyphenols are also found in fruits, vegetables, tea, and olive oil.

Manuka Honey, specifically, is used to inhibit the growth of helicobacter pylori the bacteria that is implicated in many stomach ulcers.

As well as these benefits, honey is also a healthier option than white sugar. Because it is a more complex sugar, you don't need to use as much of it and it is at least one quarter water. If you like the idea of honey, you could add it to herbal and fruit teas, or put a nice big dollop on top of some Greek yoghurt, for a traditional Greek dessert.

82.   Showers vs baths

A hysterectomy will make you less flexible for a few weeks, you will find it difficult to bend, and getting up and down from a chair can be a marathon. So, rather than trying to make life difficult, use the shower instead of the bath, they are so much easier to get out of.

As well as this wonderful sense of ease, it will be easier to keep any wounds and any dressings you have clean and dry.

But what happens if you don't have a shower?

Perhaps investing in a hand-held shower spray might be a good idea, at least that way you can sit on the side of the bath to wash yourself with a face cloth. If this still isn't an option and you have no choice but to use a bath then it might be worth spending a little time before your operation working out how you're going to get in and out and whether you have enough room around you to do it comfortably. You must remember not to soak any wounds or dressings in water, so keep it to a just a few inches in the bottom of the bath if that's going to be a concern.

Once any wounds have healed and you have become more flexible, then the warm water of a bath can be a wonderful way to relax, but remember don't add any bath oils or bubbles until you are healed completely; you don't want to undo all the good you've already done.

83.   Bake your own menopause cake

This is my version of a cake originally developed by Linda Kearns who was tired of taking HRT and who wanted to reduce her menopausal symptoms more naturally.

Convinced that phytoestrogens were the way forward, she formulated a recipe that would provide her with the optimal daily amount of soya and linseed. ideally you should eat one slice a day.

- ❖ 100g (4oz) soy flour
- ❖ 100g (4oz) wholewheat flour
- ❖ 1pc stem ginger finely chopped
- ❖ 100g (4oz) porridge oats
- ❖ 100g (4oz) raisins
- ❖ 1 ripe peeled banana
- ❖ 50g (2oz) sunflower seeds

- ❖ 50g (2ozg) sesame seeds
- ❖ 0g (2oz) pumpkin seeds
- ❖ 100g (4oz) linseeds

- ❖ ½ tsp ground ginger
- ❖ ½ tsp cinnamon
- ❖ ½ teaspoon nutmeg
- ❖ ¾ litre (900ml) soya milk

❖ 50g (2oz) cup flaked almonds

Put all the dry ingredients in a large mixing bowl. Add the soya milk, mix well and leave to soak for about 30 minutes. Meanwhile, heat the oven to 190°C. Line a small loaf tin with waxed paper.

Spoon the mixture into the baking tin and bake for 1½ hours. If the mixture ends up too stiff or too thick to pour, stir in some more soya milk. Test with a skewer and if it is not cooked through, allow five to ten more minutes. Turn out on a wire rack to cool. It is delicious with butter or on its own.

84.   Bowel cleansing drink

If you are having problems with constipation, perhaps because you have some pain, or fear of pain, then this is the drink for you.

❖ 1 small bottle prune juice
❖ 1 small apple, peeled, cored and chopped
❖ 1 small teaspoon linseeds
❖ ½ litre sparkling mineral water

Put all the ingredients in a blender and whiz on full power for a couple of minutes, pour into a jug and keep in the fridge for the day.

Drink a small glass in the morning, afternoon and evening, together with plenty of plain water, until it works!

In the long term

85. Banish the sweats naturally

Hot flushes and night sweats are a major symptom of the menopause which, for some women, can be unbearable and very disruptive, whilst others barely notice them and their effects. They can make you feel very self-conscious even though they often aren't noticed by anyone else.

Research has shown that a combination of Vitamin C and Bioflavonoids[17] are very effective at controlling hot flushes, and the recommended dose is between one to three grams per day. In addition, Vitamin E also seems to have a positive effect on these symptoms.

Herbal remedies are common on the shelves of health food stores and the American Indians have used Black Cohosh effectively for centuries. It has been shown to be effective in balancing female hormones as well relieving menopausal symptoms[18]. However, if you have had a hysterectomy because of cancer or endometriosis you may want to avoid it as it is one of the most oestrogenic of plants.

Yarrow has been used to lower body temperature, whilst Vitex Agnus Castus is considered one of the most potent remedies because it stimulates and balances the pituitary gland which, in turn, controls and balances our hormones: it's also good for reducing hot flushes[19].

Korean red ginseng helps overcome any depression you may feel. And, increasing your levels of phyotonutrients by increasing the amounts of fruit and vegetables you eat, can help to balance the body. Omega 3 fatty acids may help prevent post-menopausal osteoporosis, breast cancer and cardio-vascular disease.

And finally, aromatherapy massage, perhaps using sage, chamomile and lavender; seems to help some menopausal symptoms – seems like an excellent reason to indulge!

86.   Take a holiday

This holiday is elevated to a prescription for you and It's time to indulge.

What is your ideal holiday? Do you want a whole week of relaxing on a beach and lying in the sun being waited on? Or would that drive you mad because you'd far rather be out exploring. How about a combination of the two, depending on how your fatigue levels are?

It is possible that the health problems leading to your hysterectomy have impacted on your choice of holiday in the past to a greater or lesser extent. Have you thought about what it could be like to travel unrestricted and wear what you like around the pool? Have new horizons opened up that were impossible in the past?

Holidays are also a fantastic opportunity to revitalise your relationship, as they are time out from the daily routine.

If you do plan a holiday that involves travel by air or sea though, you may need to find out from your travel insurer if there are any restrictions following surgery. They can also give you guidance about when it is appropriate to travel.

87.   Give a little back

If you've done all the things suggested in this book, then one hint you might have enjoyed was spending time some on our forums talking to other women around the world who have also had a hysterectomy.

Now that you are almost recovered and have all that experience behind you, why not consider using it, for a time, to help other women who might be as concerned and nervous as you once were. Not only will it help you put your experience into perspective, but it will be a tremendous help for others.

If you did have a difficult time, talk about it and share what did, and didn't, work for you. You can almost guarantee that someone, somewhere, sometime, is going to thank you for donating those pearls of wisdom to the world.

In the same way, if you had a good experience, talk about it and shout it from the rooftops.

So, if you haven't joined the forums yet you can do so here: *www.hysterectomy-association.org.uk/contact-us/join-us/*. Alternatively, why not send us your stories to add to our 'In My Own Words' blog. Last of all, what about sending us your own hints and tips and we will add them to our free emails.

88.   Change of life or change your life?

Psychotherapists regard hysterectomy and the menopause as a major life stage for a woman. When the menopause occurs at the same time as other significant life events, it often becomes a time for reflection on the past and a rethink on where you're going.

Would you like life to stay very much as it is, or are there some things you'd like to change. Have you got things on a 'must do' list, that are undone? Have you got any dreams or passions that life and health had made impossible until now?

You've got to take it easy physically for the next few weeks, but that doesn't mean you can't use your head for planning. In your recovery journal answer the question *"what is the meaning of life"*, then have a short rest before you get started!

89.   Returning to work

If you ask a gynaecologist or doctor when you can go back to work, their stock answer is that everyone will be fine to go back after six weeks. Of course, this is dependent on many different factors and, in the experience of the Hysterectomy Association, the average length of time women take before returning to work is between nine and thirteen weeks if they have abdominal surgery.

Women having minimally invasive surgery such as a vaginal hysterectomy often return to work at between four and eight weeks. You can work out the reason for such differing timescales and your own needs by answering the following questions.

1.   What type of operation did you have? If it was minimally invasive you won't have the large wounds that also need to heal. If it was abdominal, then you're recovering from the operation as much as the removal of your womb.
2.   Why did you have a hysterectomy?
3.   How ill were you before your operation? If you have been suffering illness for the past few months or even years, you will need time to recover from this, as well as the surgery.
4.   How do you get to work, by bus, car or walking? You need to consider the fatigue factor and build up to walking or standing for that length of time.
5.   What type of work do you do? Your muscles need to recover their previous levels of fitness, standing, lifting, bending and stretching will need to be introduced gradually otherwise you run the risk of doing too much too soon.
6.   How much support you have had at home during recovery? Will you be working *and* looking after your home *and* any children? You might have other responsibilities too, caring or additional jobs and hobbies.

Women in jobs that involve standing for extended periods, or where there is a lot of lifting, stretching or bending probably need a slightly longer period of recovery may be needed. Those who have desk jobs may be able to get back to work slightly sooner.

It is advisable to talk to your employer as soon as you are given a date for your operation as they may need to find temporary replacement. You will also need to check your entitlement to sick pay. If you are a manager then it's a good idea to prepare your staff to cover for you.

And, and if you are self-employed, you will need to let your clients know you won't be around for a while.

When you do go back to work you may need to think about doing reduced hours or a different job for a few weeks. For those who really can't keep away, what about seeing if you can do some work at home.

Keeping in touch with the HR department and your line manager will keep you up to date with everything and keep them informed about how you're doing.

The key thing to remember is to be realistic about what you can, and can't, do.

90.   Managing weight gain

Weight gain after a hysterectomy seems almost inevitable, but there can be many reasons that aren't just down to surgery.

It might be that your tummy has changed shape because a major muscle (the uterus) has been removed, and you've got the classic hysterectomy pot belly. You might be bloated with wind and water retention. It's also tempting to eat your normal diet and quantities forgetting you are not doing your usual activities and therefore are using less energy than normal during recovery. Whilst it's important to eat a healthy diet as your body needs food to help fuel regeneration, comfort eating is a significant risk factor for most women, occurring mostly out of boredom.

To recover well, you need to give your body the right quantities of protein, fat and carbohydrates; as well as all the essential vitamins and minerals. If you are a calorie counter, it's important to remember that not all calories are equal and some are better for you than others. Ultimately the only way to lose weight is to use more energy than you are putting in, so a gentle increase in your daily activity levels should be very helpful.

Having said all that, you have just had a major operation and you are entitled to pamper yourself for a while, perhaps by reaching for an apple instead of a biscuit.

91.   Become a belly dancer

I know when you read this, the last thing you are going to consider is belly dancing; but belly dancing (or Raks Sharqi as it is also called) works with the body, not against it.

The graceful hip drops, rolls, and pivots use many of the muscle groups in the abdomen, pelvis, trunk, spine, and neck and of course such movements come naturally to the female form.

When you're feeling better and looking for some gentle exercise, it could be worth finding out if there is a local class. The movements will tone the muscles and help maintain your flexibility in a safe and effective way. It can also help prevent lower back problem, tone up your arms and shoulders and, as it is weight bearing, help to prevent osteoporosis.

As well as all these benefits, you can burn anywhere between 250 and 300 calories an hour at a class because it is a fast dance. So if you have some extra weight to shift then this could be the exercise for you. But, before you do anything, check with your GP that it's okay for you to start, you don't want to overdo it now do you?

92.   Try Tai Chi, Yoga or Pilates

Like belly dancing, Tai Chi, Yoga and Pilates are all exercises that work on with your inner core. You can start all of them just a few months after your hysterectomy as they are very gentle, don't require you to push yourself too far too fast and will help you tone up and regain vitality and flexibility. In fact, they are perfect for beginners at exercise, as well as those recovering from surgery.

Classes focus on moving the body slowly through a series of precise movements while concentrating on your breathing as you are doing them.

Because the movements are so specific, teachers concentrate on making sure you do them correctly ensuring you place as little strain as possible on joints and muscles which prevents injury. Committing to attend a regular class will help you relax and improve stamina, coordination, breathing, concentration, strength, body alignment and general fitness.

Before you start a class though, you should let the teacher know that when you had your operation so they can take it into account when asking you to do the movements.

93.   Getting behind the steering wheel

Some hospital information leaflets recommend you wait six weeks after an abdominal hysterectomy before you try driving again. Some will vary the timescale according to the type of hysterectomy you had, with less invasive forms of surgery naturally having an earlier timescale to work to.

However, you're the expert on your body and there are five things to consider, together with any other general recommendations made by the hospital.

❖ You may be surprised by how your much you use your abdominal muscles when driving;

❖ You need to be able to use the clutch, accelerator and brake, if you can't do this your insurance is invalid;

❖ You must be able to do an emergency stop without hesitation, if you can't do this your insurance is invalid;

❖ Check the requirements of your insurance policy and notify them if required to do so;

❖ You must be able to turn your head to see behind you for reversing.

If you are happy with all the above, try yourself in a parked car first and then keep your excursions brief the first few times you go out. It's also helpful to take a friend who can also drive with you, just in case you don't feel able to get home again.

94. All about sex

You're unique, did you know that? Although the hospital leaflet may have suggested you refrain from sex for six weeks, only you will know whether the time is right. At around the six-week mark, there should be no pain in your genitals or abdomen, any external wounds you have should have healed, and any internal wounds should be well on their way to full recovery; discharge should have stopped and you could feel emotionally ready. Sex before this time risks infection, regardless of the type of surgery you had. It could also pull away any internal stitching.

Preparing for the big moment is important; after all you may have associated sex with discomfort and pain for some time before your hysterectomy. But now this is the new you.

Set the scene with warmth and no interruptions. Use a room fragrance such as ylang-ylang and turn down the lights. Add some massage oil to get you in the mood and add the gift of time, lots of it.

Let your partner make sure you are well lubricated, either naturally or with KY Jelly, and enjoy. If you're worried about the depth of penetration or anticipate pain, then girls on top might be a treat for both of you, allowing too feel comfortable and stay in control. Afterwards, cuddle up close and make plans for your new life ahead.

95.   Treat yourself to a day spa

You are finally about to go back to work and feeling pretty good considering, although you've spent a lot of time alone doing not very much, you could really do with just one more bit of 'me' time now you're feeling fit and well.

If you can afford it, book yourself into a local spa for the day and indulge in a massage, a facial, tasty food and relaxation away from the world with a book.

If you can't head out to a spa, why not create one at home instead.

The first thing to do is remove your responsibilities; if you have children, persuade someone to have them for you for the day or collect them from school; make sure your partner is at work and book yourself in for a haircut. You could get a manicure and pedicure done at the same time.

Once home light some candles in the bathroom, run a warm bath and add some delicious bath oils to soften the skin and put on some relaxing music (just loud enough for you to hear in the bathroom).

Finally close the blinds, draw the curtains, turn the lights out, or down, and slip into the bath and lie quietly for an hour or so. When you get out, dry yourself off and rub in plenty of body lotion.

Wrap yourself up in a bathrobe and settle down on the sofa with a glass of wine and your favourite book or film; bliss. Who knows, you may even make this a regular event.

96.   Burn the tampons

A woman once wrote to me saying on her trips to the supermarket she would skip past the sanitary towel aisle, safe in the knowledge she wouldn't have to go through anything like that again.

Being creative with how you dispose of your remaining sanitary products and contraceptives is one way of demonstrating the very powerful change you have experienced through your hysterectomy; change for the better for most women.

Since you hit puberty your body has been ruled by hormones, your period pains and bleeding as well as all the other symptoms that led you to the point of having a hysterectomy. Well, it's time to let go of all the negative stuff and look forward to the future.

You are no longer tied to your periods, life isn't limited, there is nothing to stop you abseiling down the front of the office building or leaping out of a plane at 10,000 feet if you really want to. The sky is your limit and you can enjoy the life you were always meant to have.

What about hosting a barbeque and use your spare tampons and pads as briquettes, or build a bonfire. Either way, using fire to say 'out with the old' is extremely symbolic.

Alternatively, you could do something fun, like making a tampon angel if it's close to Christmas, just search online for instructions; Why not get your girlfriends in and have a party of it with some wine and nibbles; at the very least you'll have a laugh. (P.S. I'd recommend dipping the tampons in water and hanging them up by the string the day before the party).

If none of these are for you, or if you have huge stocks, why not donate them to your local women's refuge or food bank.

Now, every time you go to your local supermarket, glide down the sanitary towel aisle saying to yourself "thank you for the extra days I have every month".

97.   Take care of your heart health

More women die of heart disease and its related illnesses such as stroke and other cardiovascular diseases than any other illness. And more young women die of heart disease than cancer.

If you have a hysterectomy that removes your ovaries, the reduction in oestrogen, thought to be help protect women against heart disease, means you need to look after your heart. Together with your bone health, your heart is directly affected by the menopause.

For women who keep their ovaries but go on to experience an early menopause, the same recommendation applies.

One option is to take HRT, if you are interested you will need to speak to your GP. If you don't want to do this, changing your diet and lifestyle can be beneficial. Check out the following as a useful starting point. Later you can head online to the British Heart Foundation at *www.hriuk.org* for more hints and tips.

❖ Increase the levels of Vitamin C, Vitamin E, Vitamin D and essential fatty acids, beta-carotene by taking a good quality supplement.

❖ Add Ginkgo biloba, hawthorn, garlic and ginger as supplements or through diet and herbal teas.

❖ Take regular aerobic exercise, something that increases your heart rate for 30 minutes at least three times a week.

❖ Balance your intake of healthy fats, high quality protein and carbohydrates.

❖ Eat more fruit, vegetables, nuts, whole grains and seeds.

98.   Look after your skin and hair

Ageing affects the skin and hair noticeably. We all get wrinkles on our face; more grey hairs appear every year and having major surgery will show up here as well.

The menopause can precipitate skin and hair ageing; and both your skin and hair may become drier and more fragile.

Using a moisturiser and a good sunscreen to prevent prolonged exposure to the sun will help your skin; and conditioning treatments especially for dry hair will help keep its lustre.

You can also eat your way to good skin and hair, by including plenty of eggs and liver for Vitamin A; dark green leafy vegetables, sweet potatoes and carrots for beta carotene; vegetable oils, nuts and seeds for your essential fatty acids and shellfish, red meat and pumpkin seeds for zinc.

As well as a healthy diet, drinking plenty of water will ensure that your skin looks full and plump and help your hair to be less dry and brittle.

You can also try one of the following natural remedies every couple of months or so.

❖   Mix 2 tablespoons of honey and 2 teaspoons of whole milk. Smooth over your face and throat. Relax, perhaps in a warm bath, for 15 minutes before rinsing off with warm water. Finally, splash your face with cold water to reinvigorate it.

❖ To give your hair a real shine; dissolve 1 teaspoon of honey into a large glass of warm water and use as a hair rinse. If you're blonde, add the juice of 1 lemon as well. Rinse well with warm water

99. Plan a recovery party

So how are you going to celebrate the new liberated you?

That's you with the new life, new image and new positive outlook. What about celebrating with a recovery party to say thanks to everyone that has helped you on the way to health?

All those people who have done the dishes, got the shopping and been there to talk to and cry with.

Celebrate your success with a cake and sparkling wine. You could even spend some of your recovery time thinking about the message you would like on the top of your cake; will it be funny or thought provoking?

So, get your friends to bring the food, ask the supermarket to deliver the drinks, persuade everyone to bring their own glasses and plates (so you don't have to wash up) and have fun, celebrating your health and happiness.

100. Get a grip on your bones

After going through the menopause, whether surgically because they were removed or because they fail early, you may have an increased risk of osteoporosis as your hormone levels change over the next few years.

One way of monitoring the strength of your bones is by regular (every three to five years) bone mineral densitometry tests your GP can arrange for you. This scan will spot potentially harmful changes to your bone strength meaning appropriate action can be taken.

You can also help yourself by taking moderate, regular bone strengthening exercise such as walking or running, and by changing to dietary habits that contribute to your bone health:

* Increase your levels of Vitamin D, calcium, magnesium and boron;
* Eat dark green leafy vegetables, fruit, whole grains and seeds;
* Add oily fish, baked beans and dried fruit to your diet;
* Avoid having too much red meat and coffee
* And if you smoke, stop.

101. Dance

The author and artist Vivian Greene once said, "Life is not about waiting for the storm to pass...it's about learning how to dance in the rain!".

True dance, the kind unfettered by convention, breaks the rules and shares joy that comes from within, is a powerful personal expression of the woman you have become. It is a simple way to reconnect with the younger you; the rebellious teenager, the partying twenty-something you were before the health issues set in and the rules of society dictated how you were supposed to 'be'.

Ecstatic dance, fully conscious free form dance, allows you the freedom to move your body in ways that feel most expressive and comfortable for you and perfect for everyone who loves to dance when no-one else is watching.

But it's also so much more than movement to music; dancing in self-expression gives you permission to be angry, happy, sad and joyful all at the same time. It releases endorphins, those feel good hormones that lift the spirits; and gives you a surge of adrenaline making you feel truly alive.

So, move the furniture, roll back the rug, hire a hall or go into the garden with your favourite tunes and re-learn what it is to be, the unique, the wonderful, YOU!

Appendices

You can request a set of these appendices plus other useful resources to print out yourself by sending an email to: *resources@hysterectomy-association.org.uk.*

You will also get these appendices and much more in one of our hysterectomy recovery journals, see our online shop for more information.

For even more handy hints and tips for a happy hysterectomy visit:

www.hysterectomy-association.org.uk

Scaling Diary

Day: ..../ Date: .... / Time: ....

(1 is the worst you've had or done and 10 is the best you've had or done)

Pain	1	2	3	4	5	6	7	8	9	10
Sleeping	1	2	3	4	5	6	7	8	9	10
Mood	1	2	3	4	5	6	7	8	9	10
Tiredness	1	2	3	4	5	6	7	8	9	10
Exercise	1	2	3	4	5	6	7	8	9	10
Comments:										

Day: ..../ Date: .... / Time: ....

(1 is the worst you've had or done and 10 is the best you've had or done)

Pain	1	2	3	4	5	6	7	8	9	10
Sleeping	1	2	3	4	5	6	7	8	9	10
Mood	1	2	3	4	5	6	7	8	9	10
Tiredness	1	2	3	4	5	6	7	8	9	10
Exercise	1	2	3	4	5	6	7	8	9	10
Comments:										

Scaling Diary

Day: ..../ Date: .... / Time: ....

(1 is the worst you've had or done and 10 is the best you've had or done)

Pain	1	2	3	4	5	6	7	8	9	10
Sleeping	1	2	3	4	5	6	7	8	9	10
Mood	1	2	3	4	5	6	7	8	9	10
Tiredness	1	2	3	4	5	6	7	8	9	10
Exercise	1	2	3	4	5	6	7	8	9	10
Comments:										

Day: ..../ Date: .... / Time: ....

(1 is the worst you've had or done and 10 is the best you've had or done)

Pain	1	2	3	4	5	6	7	8	9	10
Sleeping	1	2	3	4	5	6	7	8	9	10
Mood	1	2	3	4	5	6	7	8	9	10
Tiredness	1	2	3	4	5	6	7	8	9	10
Exercise	1	2	3	4	5	6	7	8	9	10
Comments:										

Step by Step to Recovery

Week 1	No household tasks at all
	Lie on (or in) bed as much as necessary
	Sleep when you need to
	Do as many light exercises as possible
	Shower daily
	Walk around the house and garden 2-3 times every day
	Lie down, rather than sit
	Sit, rather than stand
	Boil just enough water for a mug in a kettle
Week 2	Lie on (or in) the bed as much as necessary
	Rest for at least two hours per day
	Avoid prolonged periods of sitting or standing
	Help with washing up/drying dishes, sit down if necessary
	Sit down to prepare vegetables
	Start taking a daily 10-minute walk
	Walk around the house and garden 2-3 times daily
	Boil enough water for 2 mugs in the kettle
Week 3	Increase your daily walk by 2 minutes every day
	Use the stairs at home 2-3 times a day
	Light magazine or newspaper shopping in local area

	If you have any pain – stop immediately
	You should be able to go out in the car comfortably now
Week 4	Start walking up to 20 minutes twice a day
	Make tea and coffee for three or four people
	Help with dusting
Week 5 onwards	Start doing light routine housework
	Drive a car when you can do an emergency stop
	Can possibly use an upright vacuum cleaner
	Try gentle pelvic floor exercises – stop if you feel pain
	Try vacuuming with a cylinder cleaner (week 6-7)
	Try bed making (but not changing duvets)

Exercises for Recovery

There are a variety of exercises you can try for different stages of your recovery, I have grouped them here to make it easier to see what you should be doing and when.

Exercises for Hospital	These exercises are designed to get your circulation moving and your muscles mobile again. They can all be done in bed, but remember if you feel too much pain – then you should stop. They are similar to exercises you might do when flying to help guard against DVT.
	Roll the ankles round in a circle curling your feet towards you stretching your feet away from you Breath in deeply for a count of five and breath out slowly for a count of five
	Increase the number of times you do each of these as you feel stronger.

Week 1 – 4	Carry on with the hospital exercises whenever you are lying on the bed.
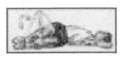	Lie on your back with your knees bent up, as if you were going to get out of bed. Allow the knees to drop first to one side, and then to the other.

Lie on your back with your knees bent up and press the middle of your back down into the mattress by pulling in your tummy muscles as hard as you can at this stage, tighten your buttocks at the same time. Hold as long as you can and then release.

Lie on your back with your knees resting on a pillow and your arms by your sides. Now gently stretch one arm towards your feet along the side of your body and then come back; repeat on the other side,

Gradually increase the number of times you do each of these exercises as your muscles get stronger. |

Weeks 5 - 7 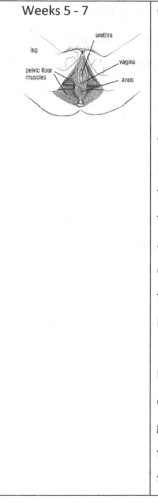	Carry on with all the exercises listed in the previous weeks, increasing the number of repetitions you are doing daily. Introduce Pelvic Floor Exercises. To locate the right muscles, next time you are on the loo, tighten your abdominal muscles so that the flow or urine stops. Count up to five and then release the flow. The aim is to prevent any leakage at all. You can repeat these exercises as much as your muscles are able to as they will help prevent possible future incontinence or prolapse. Improve your abdominal muscles by lying on your back with your knees bent and then gently lift your head and shoulders off the floor (or bed) and reach your hands down towards your knees.

References

1. Originally published on 'Songs by Tom Lehrer', 1953

2. http://ash.org.uk/information-and-resources/briefings/briefing-smoking-and-surgery/ and http://www.quit.org.au/about/frequently-asked-questions/how-does-smoking-affect-my-body/smoking-and-surgery.html

3. The International Aloe Science, Council

4. http://www.iasc.org/articles.html

5. Parker, W.H. & Parker, L. A Gynaecologists Second Opinion, 1996; p275

6. Celso-Ramon Garcia, M.D. Winnifred B. Cutler, Ph.D. Preservation of the Ovary: A Re-evaluation, Fertility and Sterility (Vol.42. No.4 October, 1984)

7. Parker, W.H. & Parker, L. A Gynaecologists Second Opinion, 1996; p277

8. Goldfarb, H.A. & Greif, J. The No Hysterectomy Option, 1997, pp147-148

9. Davis, S.R. The use of testosterone after menopause, J Br Menopause Soc 2004 Jun;10(2): pp65-9

10. Prasad A.S. et al, Zinc status and serum testosterone levels of healthy adults, Nutrition. 1996 May;12(5):344-8

11. Ernst E. The benefits of Arnica: 16 case reports, Homeopathy 2003 Oct;92(4): pp217-9

12. Lydeking-Olsen E. et al, Soymilk or progesterone for prevention of bone loss--a 2 year randomized, placebo-controlled trial, Eur J Nutr 2004 Aug;43(4): pp246-57

13. Seeger H. et al, The effect of progesterone and synthetic progestins on serum- and estradiol-stimulated proliferation of human breast cancer cells, Horm Metab Res 2003 Feb;35(2): pp76-80.

14. EA Hoge et al. The effect of mindfulness meditation training on biological acute stress responses in generalized anxiety disorder Psychiatry Res, 2017, http://www.psy-journal.com/article/S0165-1781(16)30847-2/fulltext

15. Sandoval M. et al, Anti-inflammatory and antioxidant activities of cat's claw (Uncaria tomentosa and Uncaria guianensis) are independent of their alkaloid content, Phytomedicine 2002 May;9(4): pp325-37

16. Philp HA. Hot flashes--a review of the literature on alternative and complementary treatment approaches, Altern Med Rev 2003 Aug;8(3): pp284-302

17. Viereck V. et al, Black cohosh: just another phytoestrogen?, Trends Endocrinol Metab 2005 May 28.

18. AJJ Van den Berg et al. An in vitro examination of the antioxidant and anti-inflammatory properties of buckwheat honeyJournal of wound care Volume 17, No 4 April 2008

19. Chopin Lucks B. Vitex agnus castus essential oil and menopausal balance: a research update, Complement Ther Nurs Midwifery 2003 Aug;9(3): pp157-60.

Bibliography

Charlish, A. Cleansing for Body and Spirit, 2000, Haldane Mason Ltd

Clark, J. Hysterectomy and the Alternatives, Vermillion, 2000

Costantino, M. The Detox Handbook, 2003, S Webb and Son

Davis, P. Aromatherapy An A-Z, 1996, CW Daniel Company Limited

DeAngelo, D. Sudden Menopause, 2001, Newleaf

Gray, D. Fresh Smoothies, 2000, Chancellor Press

Glenville, M, Natural Alternatives to HRT, Kyle Cathie, 1997

Glenville, M. and Esson L. Natural Alternatives to HRT Cookbook, 2000, Kyle Cathie

Glenville, M. and Esson, L. Healthy Eating for the Menopause, 2004, Kyle Cathie

Glouberman, Dr D., Life Choices, Life Changes, 2003, Hodder and Stoughton

Goldfarb H.A. and Greif, J. The No-Hysterectomy Option, 1997, Wiley

Hay, L. You Can Heal Your Life, Hay House, 1984

Lerner, H.G. The Dance of Intimacy, 1989, Harper Collins

McWhirter, A. and Clasen, L. (ed) Foods that Harm, foods that heal, 2002, Readers Digest

Merson, S. Lift Off, 100 Tips to Energize, 2003, MQ Publications

Miller, J. Guide to Reflexology, 2000, Caxton Editions

Parker, W. and Parker, R,L. A Gynaecologists Second Opinion, Plume/Penguin 1996

Parkinson-Hardman, L. The Pocket Guide to Hysterectomy, 2005, The Hysterectomy Association

Richardson, R. Natural Superwoman, 2003, Kyle Cathie

Robinson, Dr A. The Which Guide to Womens Health, 1996, Which Consumer Guides

Sexual Health (ed), 2002, Geddes and Grossett

Shealy C.N. (ed) The Compete Illustrated Encycolpeida of Alternative Healing Therapies, Element, 1999

Shepperson Mills, D. and Vernon, M. Endometriosis, A key to healing through nutrition, 1999, Element Books Limited

Simester, L. The Natural Health Bible, 2001, Quadrille Publishing

Tosh, C. Guide to Meditation, 2001, Caxton Editions

Webb, A. Hysterectomy a new horizon (leaflet)

Womens Health, (ed) 2000, Geddes and Grosset

Do you need more?

I would like to invite you to continue your search for relevant information by joining on our website: *www.hysterectomy-association.org.uk*

❖ Share your worries, concerns and triumphs with other women

❖ Read the blog to find out more about the latest research

❖ Get the latest information about the alternatives that may be appropriate

❖ Join us and get lots of extra member benefits as well as knowing that you are helping many other women in the future benefit too

❖ Join us on Facebook www.*facebook.com/HysterectomyUK*

❖ Follow us on Twitter *@HysterectomyUK*

If you would like Linda to come and speak to your organisation or group, please contact the Hysterectomy Association by sending an email to *info@hysterectomy-association.org.uk*

More books on Amazon:

- ❖ In My Own Words: Women's experience of hysterectomy - *http://amzn.to/2qSmLuV*
- ❖ Losing the Woman Within - *http://amzn.to/2qT3O9b*
- ❖ The Pocket Guide to Hysterectomy - *http://amzn.to/2qh828K*
- ❖ Hysteria 1 – *http://amzn.to/2reaphB*
- ❖ Hysteria 2 – *http://amzn.to/2qhgdlo*
- ❖ Hysteria 3 – *http://amzn.to/2qTprGN*
- ❖ Hysteria 4 – *http://amzn.to/2q8pwZT*
- ❖ Hysteria 5 – *http://amzn.to/2qTfPeM*

More books from Linda Parkinson-Hardman on Amazon:

- ❖ Woman on the Edge of Reality - *http://amzn.to/2q8chIt*
- ❖ LinkedIn Made Easy – *http://amzn.to/2qhbTCL*
- ❖ Selling Online: A beginner's guide - *http://amzn.to/2rebWEf*
- ❖ A Diva's Guide to the Menopause - *http://amzn.to/2rNpBP*

Made in United States
North Haven, CT
18 April 2023